NO MORE
FEARS

Also by Douglas Hunt

NO MORE CRAVINGS

Douglas Hunt, M.D.

NO MORE FEARS

WARNER BOOKS

A Warner Communications Company

Library of Congress Cataloging-in-Publication Data

Hunt, Douglas, 1930–
  No more fears.

  Bibliography: p.
  Includes index.
  1. Phobias. 2. Anxiety. I. Title.
RC535.H86   1988   616.85'225   87-21702
ISBN 0-446-51361-X

Designed by Giorgetta Bell McRee

To Norma, Dick, Steve and Ginny
with love

CONTENTS

NO MORE
FEARS

PART

1

GETTING READY TO CHANGE

INTRODUCTION

The cold steel blade of the scissors glistened in her upraised hand. One blade swung across the other, forming a cross, their target— Berri's neck—only inches away. She trembled as she twisted her head to the side to bare the raised line of her jugular and checked it in the mirror. Her arm cocked upward again for the lethal thrust. A thought screamed at her, Now—do it—now! Berri braced herself for the pain. One stroke and it would be all over. All the dark foreboding that choked and froze her windpipe, all the horror that haunted her.

A slight hesitation was enough to weaken her resolve. The scissors fell from her hand, and she collapsed to the floor on her knees, sobbing. Everything seemed so futile, so hopeless, so meaningless. Depression and fear tore at her. Pain was everywhere.

As she rocked back and forth in grief, she bumped against the coffee table, spilling the contents of her purse. Amid the paraphernalia strewn on the floor was a small bottle of pills. Impulsively, she grabbed the capsules and devoured them without water. They were bitter, but she stoically chewed and swallowed. I had given her the pills earlier in the week, just in case an "attack" should occur. She had finally remembered to take them.

Berri now fought to slow down her thoughts. It wasn't easy, for her mind wouldn't behave. She continued to rock back and forth and moan as she struggled to understand what was happening. As the moments passed, she found it increasingly difficult to recall exactly why she had wanted to die. When her emotions subsided, she began to wonder why she was even considering suicide. And why was she crouched on the floor like some kind of madwoman? The torment was now draining out of her; and when the last vestiges of horrific emotion receded, she felt a tremendous sense of relief. It was over.

Berri had come to my office seeking help in coping with severe anxiety, depression, and phobias. After some preliminary testing, we discovered she had cerebral allergic reactions to certain foods, which could trigger catastrophic panic attacks. She was especially susceptible to the food grains in alcohol; drinking set off bouts of paranoia and irrational thinking. The biochemical reaction also caused her face and body to turn beet red. Her mother had experienced the same flushing when she drank alcohol but suffered only minor psychological symptoms.

In view of Berri's history, I prescribed a combination of nutritional supplements for her to keep near her at all times in case of an allergic attack. On this particular night, my patient had been in a mood to celebrate. She had gone to a Chinese restaurant with friends and had ordered four alcoholic drinks in rapid succession. While in the restaurant, she had become increasingly belligerent and finally walked out in a huff, leaving her friends embarrassed and bewildered. Her driving was erratic; and when she got home and looked in the mirror, she discovered that her face was a deep scarlet. Her hysteria quickly evolved from there. Fortunately the nutritional supplements terminated the attack before Berri made a serious attempt on her life.

NORMAL vs. ABNORMAL FEARS

Every one of us will, at certain times, experience general anxiety, as well as specific fears. Can you honestly imagine not feeling terror during a high-magnitude earthquake or while looking down from one of the top floors of a skyscraper? Such fears are rational and perfectly normal. Some people, on the other hand, develop fears that most of us would consider unreasonable because they are caused by no real or present danger. Classified as *phobias*, these include fears of everything from shoes to shopping centers. The common denominator is that their origins are irrational rather than reasonable. They are often exaggerated responses to conditions in our society. To understand them, we must look at the world in which we live.

Stressful Society

Life has never been easy or without dangers. Even primitive tribes suffered some forms of stress. Survival meant defending themselves against nature, wild animals, and hostile enemies. Yet, in spite of all the difficulties experienced in primitive environments, our ancestors seem to have exhibited much less anxiety than their modern descendants. Perhaps they were simply too busy hunting and protecting the home front to spend much time dwelling on emotions. Their goals were simple and fundamental; all their energies were focused on sheer survival.

Faced with the problems of a rapidly changing society, we are also confronted with financial and career uncertainties, social and political concerns, and anxieties over health and relationships. Just being alive can sometimes be a pretty scary thing. Throughout history, philosophers have struggled with the concept of how man manages to endure the knowledge of his limited and vulnerable existence. Besides the ever-increasing sources of our personal stresses, we are bombarded daily by television, radio, and the press with the national and international crises that threaten our existence. The precarious state of our environment is brought home when we hear about acid rain, radon gas in our homes, and toxic waste dumps. Each one of these concerns is significant cause for worry, and together they represent an overwhelming load.

The manufacture and widespread distribution of chemicals has already had a profound effect on our psychological as well as our physical health. Those of us in the mental-health field have long recognized their potential danger to the brain. Researchers have observed the increased occurrence of depression, anger, anxiety, and thinking disturbances due to common chemicals found in our environment, such as formaldehyde and phenols.

The ultimate result of all this is a dramatic rise in the incidence of stress and anxiety. Thousands more succumb each day to anxiety-induced disease. And for all the cases reported, many others go undiagnosed. No one knows what the ultimate outcome will be. It is now an accepted fact that over 100 million Americans are significantly depressed. Attempts have been made to reverse this trend by utilizing psychological approaches, but they have clearly not been effective or the problem would be disappearing.

Prescription drugs for anxiety and depression are not a sufficient answer, for their side effects often prove to be as troublesome as the original symptoms. And there is another problem—these drugs can only be used for short periods of time or they will become seriously addictive, which further limits their value.

Traditionally, alcohol has been a convenient "security blanket" for many. Now it has been replaced by new recreational drugs which many people consider trendy and more exciting. Designer drugs seem, as some users like to say, "fresh."

The amazing thing is that those turning to drugs range from cowboys and carpenters to doctors, lawyers, teachers, stockbrokers, and even those holding high office. Headlines used to reveal scandals involving prosecuting attorneys who took drugs just as the felons in their courtroom did, but today such news is no longer even startling.

It seems that the need for chemical escape is universal. A growing number of research studies now show that the underlying cause of drug abuse is based not on a simple desire for hedonistic kicks, but on a compelling need to relieve depression and anxiety. These emotions are painful, and often the pain is greater than many people can bear.

As we stand and watch the foundation of our society being fractured and torn apart by drug abuse, it's clear that the effects of stress are at an almost unmanageable level and present-day answers are not stemming the tide. In the war against drugs, the underlying causes are unfortunately being ignored. Nutritional approaches are not the total answer to combating stress and anxiety, but they can be a powerful tool in reversing the desperate needs that many of us have to escape into drugs and alcohol.

THE BENEFITS OF THIS BOOK

This book is about "normal" anxieties as well as "abnormal" fears. Often it can be difficult to separate the two. I will explore the differences between abnormal or pathological fears and common everyday anxieties, and discuss ways to deal with each of them effectively. If a particular fear has ever kept you from experiencing pleasure, or in any way interferes with your personal or career potential, then it can and should be brought under control.

As one astute observer has said, "There is an enormous gap between advice and help." In the past, most authorities pushed psychological *advice* for the control of anxiety and fear, and the bulk of that advice was not even new information. This book is unique in that it offers real help in the form of significant and immediate relief. The approach I recommend is biological treatment with vitamins, minerals, amino acids, and improved nutrition.

In *No More Fears* we'll deal with the broad spectrum of anxiety —everything from the most severe agoraphobia all the way down to simple shyness. In between, I'll cover nightmares, daymares, fear of flying, fear of exams, fear of public speaking, business worries, fear of AIDS, and so on. If you have a fear that you want to control, chances are this book will have the answer.

The relief of fear through nutritional supplements can be quick and easy, but it is not possible to avoid fear altogether. Fear can only really be conquered by facing it head-on. This book also contains coping techniques and desensitization methods which can be used along with the nutritional supplements. In addition, I'll discuss the pros and cons of the anxiety-reducing drugs commonly prescribed by physicians. There are obviously many approaches that can be used in controlling fear. This book focuses on self-control, not by using the mind alone, but by making use of nature's chemicals—the essential ingredients that can help you correct your own biochemical imbalances.

Is Self-Help a Workable Solution?

Can forms of self-help produce a viable solution to anxiety and fear disorders? Research is affirmative (Phillips and Johnson 1972). Although working with a trained professional is generally considered preferable, self-therapy definitely has value. In the Phillips-Johnson study, 50 percent of those who relied on self-help programs rated themselves "cured" or "greatly improved," and none of the people in the program said they were not helped at all, or that their condition had worsened. This is an interesting point because some therapist-oriented programs have reported adverse results.

My own experiences with self-help have been extremely positive. I had finished medical school and was a practicing psychiatrist before I fully realized what a significant role anxiety played in my life. I never knew, for example, why I was extremely shy, or why, when I became upset, I was totally unable to function. I often wondered why I felt "trapped" in crowds and in closed places and recognized that these feelings had a limiting effect on my life. Although I could explain these sensations in psychological terms, I never really felt I could control them satisfactorily.

My personal growth did not occur until I had first paid a terrible price for my ignorance. I tried medication, but like many others, I found my hypersensitivity to drugs ruled out that option and left me in a quandary. I was stuck with my anxiety and had no effective way of dealing with it. I tried relaxation and other coping techniques but, because of my demanding schedule, found them to be of limited value. Since I had a special interest in nutrition, I finally sought relief through that approach. It took quite a while, but I eventually found formulas that worked for me and have since helped thousands of my patients. Now I'm going to share them with you.

Two benefits of nutritional supplements are the relative speed with which they work and the fact that they produce few side effects. This easy method of regaining control over destructive emotions can sometimes shorten or eliminate the need for traditional and expensive long-term therapy.

Can Nutrition Help the Anxious/Fearful Person?

My experiences with the nutritional treatment of anxiety and fear convince me that it does indeed work. Volumes of literature now substantiate the value of nutritional supplements in combating depression. Many doctors believe that depression may be an underlying factor in the occurrence of anxiety, and part of such reasoning is that antidepressant medication has been used successfully in phobic patients. But regardless of that relationship, it has been proven that nutritional supplements greatly benefit most patients with mood disorders, so it is quite logical to see them benefiting victims of anxiety and fear.

Goals for This Book

The goal of this book is to give you new and valuable information with which to manage the fears and anxieties affecting your life. Through the use of proper nutrition and special nutritional supplementation, one can learn to prevent or inhibit anxieties, both rational and irrational.

The best way to approach this book is to read the first few chapters of general material in order to gain an understanding of how and why the supplements will work for you. Especially useful are the chapters on nutrition and general therapy. After reading this basic information, turn to the chapter that most interests you. For example, if your knees buckle when you speak in public, you will learn how to deal with that problem by reading the chapter on business fears. If you have an irrational fear involving closed places such as elevators, then you should read the material on claustrophobia.

Some coping strategies and formulas appear in chapters not directly related to your specific needs, but some of them may still be adapted to your problem. By exploring all of the material in the book thoroughly, you will eventually find the best possible solution. It may be that all you will ever need are a few specific vitamins, minerals, and amino acids.

I myself continue to use my "Fear Formulas," and so do members of my family—because they work. Many of my patients have gained complete control over their anxieties simply by using the correct formulas for their particular phobia. Even when this approach doesn't provide complete relief, it can at least contribute substantially to any other therapy that is being used concurrently (psychotherapy, drugs, etc.). I am sure you will benefit from the recommendations in this book as you discover the real bases for your fears along with practical and constructive ways of dealing with them.

1

Uncontrolled Fears and You

PERSONAL FEELINGS

Feelings are private property. We can try to tell others what we experience, but there is always something lost in translation. Other than measuring heart rate and blood pressure, or observing facial and behavioral changes, there is no way to measure accurately what another person is really going through. While most of us are pretty good at determining the *type* of emotion someone else is experiencing, it's harder to empathize with those feelings. For example, if one woman suffers from premenstrual syndrome (PMS) and another does not, the individual free of the disorder may complain that she doesn't understand why her friend is acting so strangely. However, when normally nonanxious patients experience anxiety as the after-effect of taking a drug, they suddenly begin to understand. "If this is the way anxious people feel," they say, "I can understand why they get so upset." Or, "If I didn't know that this nervousness was drug-induced, I'd think I was going crazy."

In addition to the problem of one person often not understanding another's feelings, a dilemma exists because people describe their emotions in different ways. For example, if drug-induced anxiety is created in normally anxiety-free individuals, they may complain about being uncomfortable or distressed and yet not feel the same sense of mortal danger that chronically anxious patients do. As a result of environment and/or genetics, some individuals are more predisposed to respond to triggering situations with anxiety and fear.

Fear vs. Anxiety—Is There a Difference?

Basically, there is no difference, and in this book I use the terms interchangeably. Arguments have been raised about this subject, but most authors consider fear and anxiety to be synonymous terms.

WHAT IS THE ANATOMY OF ANXIETY?

Anxiety is a physical reaction that occurs when one is under some kind of stress (emotional, physical, or chemical). The stress can occur without the presence of actual danger in situations such as making a speech or driving home slowly in rush-hour traffic, or it can result from exposure to truly perilous activities. Whatever the cause, real or unreal, once anxiety is initiated, it must be controlled. Even small amounts of anxiety accelerate our breathing, induce perspiration, and produce a mild sense of uneasiness. If the anxiety increases, our hearts will beat still harder and faster, our stomachs may begin to feel queasy, and muscle tension can result. At this point, anxiety may escalate into outright fear, and one might feel an overwhelming need to "escape." Any level beyond this is sheer terror, clinically known as "classic panic," arising from real or imagined loss of control. A sense of an impending disaster exaggerates the body's defenses. A pounding heart becomes a heart attack; threatened loss of self-control is equated with insanity.

In a normal individual, these degrees of anxiety are appropriately related to actual danger; but in people who have phobias, responses are completely irrational. Logic is discounted when walking through a shopping mall or seeing a kitten can suddenly make people feel as though they are having a heart attack or losing their minds. But when something in the body malfunctions, these feelings can indeed result. In light of new discoveries, such malfunctions are now known to stem not from psychological disorders, but from neurochemistry gone awry. There are a number of anatomical areas of the brain suspected of fostering this condition. Although there is currently no conclusive evidence, a growing number of researchers are giving credibility to such theories. Most experts do not believe that panic attacks are caused by overload—too much information coming in too fast for our computer brain to handle—but rather by a malfunction that originates in the body's modifiers. Whatever it is that shuts down or controls anxiety reaction is not working correctly, and thus the patient experiences "irrational" attacks of unbearable panic.

Anxiety Isn't Fun

Many things can be said about anxiety but one fact is indisputable: It's no picnic. In fact, anxiety is downright painful, a negative feeling that both humans and animals wish to avoid or escape.

Anxiety is an unpleasant feeling which has both physical and psychological components as seen below.

PHYSICAL

Altered respiration	Cold skin
Increased heart rate	Sweating
Pale skin	Weakness
Dry mouth	Trembling

PSYCHOLOGICAL

Apprehension	Awareness of pounding heart
Tension	and shortness of breath

Anxiety can be measured physically by:

Heart rate	Skin temperature
Salivary flow	EKG
Respiratory rate	Galvanic skin response

Creating Anxiety in the Lab—Further Proof of the Biological Nature of Anxiety

Adrenaline is a hormone related to the emotions of fear and rage. Injections of small amounts into the bloodstream of patients with a history of anxiety symptoms will cause those persons to experience panic attacks, while the same amount of adrenaline given to a normal individual does not produce such reactions. Such experiments prove that anxiety can easily be produced independently of psychological causes and demonstrate that abnormal anxiety can originate from biochemical disturbances without being related either to personality or to stress.

The Purpose of Anxiety

Is there any useful purpose for these anxieties and physical and psychological changes? Basically, yes. Anxiety serves as a signal that warns us of impending painful or harmful stimuli. Once warned, we can fight or flee or adjust to the problem. The rush of adrenaline that comes with anxiety gives most of us an extra edge in dealing with the adversity we are facing. On a day-to-day level, anxiety is the nag that keeps us tuned into our problems. If not excessive, it helps us get things done by not letting us become too comfortable.

Too Much Anxiety Produces
Two Problems Instead of One

When you are tense about a situation, you can actually develop two problems: the problem itself, and the need to control the attendant anxiety. Then you need not only to conquer your dilemma but also to bring your anxiety about that dilemma to a manageable level. There are many instances where, although you can't control the original situation, you can control the anxiety it produces; and that, in itself, solves part of the problem.

Anxiety Twins—Another Way to
Look at the Problem

Anxiety has two parts: a mental component and bodily tensions. Most people tackle their problems by ignoring the physical manifestations of anxiety, which they think will disappear when they figure out a way to remedy the original situation. They don't realize that the direct approach to controlling physical tensions can really be a shortcut to controlling anxiety. The direct control of anxiety is, in a very real sense, the solvable part of the problem.

In the past, therapists have utilized many techniques that quickly and successfully reduce tension. These physical approaches are both rapid and effective and can be easily learned; for example, (1) forms of exercise such as running, swimming, or biking, (2) relaxation techniques, (3) paradoxical intention, and (4) breathing control. All of these activities have a common denominator—they remove tension from the muscles, thus eliminating or reducing the level of anxiety. I will discuss each of these coping mechanisms in more depth later in the book. They can be very useful adjuncts to the nutritional supplements.

Where Does Anxiety Originate?

In addition to the physical and mental stresses listed above, we sometimes develop anxiety patterns simply by copying our parents or significant others in our early life. If these role models are nervous and tense, we too may develop similar tendencies. If they fear something in particular, such as spiders or snakes, chances are we will too. All animals learn by watching others, and humans are no exception.

Genetics also plays a significant role. At birth, we receive a body with a particular chemistry and nervous system that may or may not be stable. Some of us inherit a touchy "alarm system" that tends to go off easily. It may be "louder" than average and may not turn off as it should when it's perfectly clear that there is no real danger present. You may not like your inherited system, but you have to live with it. Since genetically programmed overreactors can be easily activated, minor threats or perceived threats can set them off. Those with touchy "alarms" can easily develop excessive fears and anxieties.

Normal People Can Develop Abnormal Fears

But what about the so-called "normal" person who suddenly develops, for example, a fear of driving? What makes this happen?

Apparently a sequence of frightening circumstances can alter the nervous system so that it becomes overly sensitive when faced with special circumstances. Soon the body becomes prone to overarousal whenever it is reexposed to those triggers.

There are a number of findings that validate this theory. Pavlov and others have induced phobias in normal laboratory animals, and research studies involving thousands of case histories have also confirmed it. There is additional historical evidence based on reports of occurrences throughout history, and, finally, demographic studies that prove the phenomenon crosses the boundaries of all races, religions, and societies.

WHAT IS AN ACTUAL PHOBIA?

A phobia is an irrational and persistent fear of a particular object, activity, or situation. A fear, however, cannot be classified as a phobia unless it causes unreasonable distress or interference with normal functioning. Phobias may originate from an unpleasant experience; often they appear without apparent cause. But telling a patient that his fears are unfounded is of no value, for the problem is not one of ignorance. Phobics know that their fears are unrealistic, and sometimes even absurd, but such facts do nothing to lessen the distress. Phobics do not imagine their fears, they *are* afraid. Such anxieties are physiologically expressed through behavior and bodily changes (trembling, withdrawal, cold hands, sweating, rapid heart rate, difficulty in breathing, and dilated pupils).

Panic attacks in any individual should not be ignored or dismissed as unimportant. They are a sign of impending difficulty. Many of these patients will eventually develop agoraphobia, the most severely disabling form of neurosis known. Such a fate is far from inevitable, however, for prompt treatment can often prevent this progression. When agoraphobia does occur, the early stages are frequently disguised as hypochondria or some other illness. Panic attacks, which seem to arise from nowhere, gradually compel the person to avoid an increasing number of activities that once comprised a normal life.

Friends and relatives often erroneously believe that patients can and should control their anxiety. This is nearly impossible to do without training, because the source of the problem is biological, not psychological. Regardless of how many attacks the patients have, they can't control their panic, since such episodes come "out of the blue," for no discernible reason. When patients realize they are powerless to stop them, they then become chronically anxious about having new attacks.

Often this condition occurs before the age of twenty, and it's not unusual for both patients and doctors to misdiagnose the malaise as a physical disorder such as a cardiac problem. Although the first attack may follow a triggering event, the attacks frequently continue to arise "on their own," unexpectedly and without warning.

If you are wondering whether or not you have phobic tendencies, even though you may not be phobic at the moment, you may want to answer the questions below to see if you have higher than average levels of fears.

FEAR PRONENESS TEST

1. Are you passive rather than assertive?
2. Do you hide your feelings (calm on the outside, but inwardly disturbed)?
3. Do you have an inordinate sense of insecurity?
4. Are you lacking in self-confidence?
5. Would you rather please others than yourself?
6. Are you unduly pessimistic and negative?
7. Are you overly imaginative, creating all sorts of horrible mental images?
8. Are you overly sensitive to other people's feelings?
9. Are you usually self-conscious, shy, and easily embarrassed?
10. Are you overly concerned with what others think about you?

If you answered yes to more than half the questions, you are more prone to fear than the average person.

OCCURRENCE OF PHOBIAS AND PANIC

Almost 15 million people in the United States suffer from phobias; one million of them can't function well enough to leave their homes.

Phobias frequently begin in early childhood, but their onset can occur at any age. Children of both genders are equally vulnerable; however, panic patients are most often females whose problems manifest themselves at about age eighteen, or at the latest, by age thirty. Phobias and panic symptoms, like all diseases, occur in varying degrees. Some individuals become openly symptomatic, while an unknown number remain subclinical and undiagnosed. Although panic and anxiety seem to occur more frequently in early adulthood and middle age, children and the elderly suffer from these problems, and many of these victims go unrecognized. A clinging child, a mama's boy or girl, who is tremendously shy and overcautious, unadventurous and abnormally conservative, may fit into this category. The elderly often show their symptoms by demanding constant attention. These oldsters sometimes select one member of the family whom they try to dominate by insisting on constant companionship and servitude.

In the one study done thus far that dealt with gender, no significant differences were found (Farley and Mealien 1981). The research investigated only one group, but it did demonstrate that there were no differences in the quantity of fear between the sexes, only in respective causes. Both males and females listed "loss of control" as their chief anxiety. Fear of failure ranked second with males, but only fourth with females. The exact opposite was true about rejection. It was number two among females, and number four among males. One of the biggest differences between the sexes was in their fear of public speaking, which was rated last by men and was third on the women's list. In general, men were more sensitive to criticism while women expressed a greater fear of animals and surgery.

The most interesting finding was that psychotic-neurotic individuals fell into about the same categories as those considered normal. The only difference was in the degree of fear. One characteristic of phobic patients was that many were hyperactive and excessively emotional during childhood. It was also noticed that many were perfectionist, hypercritical, obsessive, and often inflexible. They overreacted to the sight of blood and other fearful situations. They tended to be sensitive to their own feelings, as well as those of others, and were unduly concerned about their image, and the real or imagined difficulties of the future. These people were frequently overconscientious in an effort to please others.

About 10 percent of all patients seen in general practice have some phobic anxieties, and often this is an incidental finding. Severe fears that cause acute problems are seen in animals as well as man; from mouse to elephant, any species can become "spooked." In the human family, every culture has reported individuals with phobias, throughout the centuries. Our tendency to consider phobias a contemporary disease arising from twentieth-century stress is quickly dispelled by the ancient Greeks. They described people who, although otherwise normal, refused to leave their homes. They named these unfortunate individuals "agoraphobic," meaning those with a fear of the marketplace.

A Classification of Pathological Fears

1. **Agoraphobia**—The most severe form of all neuroses. Although it is the most commonly treated phobia, fewer patients suffer from it than from other phobic disorders. Because they fear experiencing panic attacks in a public place, true agoraphobics have great difficulty venturing outside their homes. In addition, they may also suffer from an array of other fears. Agoraphobia has accurately been described as a "fear of fear."

2. **Simple phobias**—Persistent and irrational fears of specific objects, activities, or situations. Patients usually fear only one thing and generally lead normal lives until they are faced with whatever they dread and then are overwhelmed by it.

3. **Social phobias**—Some individuals have an exaggerated fear of making fools of themselves. They may be afraid of specific activities, such as public speaking (probably one of the most universal of all fears), or may become anxious just being with people.

4. **Animal phobias**—Sufferers are usually scared of one type of animal or insect. Unless they find it impossible to avoid such creatures, they seldom feel a need to seek help.

THE TREATMENT OF FEARS

Biological psychiatry is actually closer to mainstream medicine than other branches, because it is scientific in its foundations. This approach originated in Germany and France in the mid-nineteenth century but, while striving to attain scientific validation, lost ground to Freud's psychoanalytical theories, which seemed new, fresh, and fraught with promise. Compared to his teachings, lobotomies, hydrotherapies, and electroshock seemed harsh and insensitive, and such treatments fell out of favor.

Freud's approach served to illuminate the problems of phobics and brought the subject to the forefront. It did not, however, offer a viable solution to the dilemma, and disappointing results were obtained through psychoanalysis. It was valuable for people to understand the cause of their fears, but such knowledge did not relieve their suffering. Psychotherapy is still practiced today, but has not produced much better results. For the next thirty years, until the early 1950s, other psychological approaches grew in number and diversity.

Behavioral therapy, which originated in the 1950s, called for patients to imagine themselves in fearful situations. Through this frequent confrontation using imagery, the patient theoretically gradually becomes desensitized to the subject of his fears. Direct confrontation of fears has proved infinitely more beneficial. This technique works well, but is not so effective that it cannot be improved upon. Drug therapy for phobics became available in the 1970s, with antidepressant medication achieving a high degree of success. Although phobias relate more to anxiety than to depression, the antidepressants seemed to have a significantly positive effect. The development of psychopharmacological agents, such as Librium and Valium, triggered a resurgence of interest in the biological-biochemical approach to mental disorders.

Although biological psychiatrists are still in the minority, they are gaining credence, primarily because they can now offer scientific evidence for both their diagnosis and methods of treatment. With all our wealth of information regarding neurochemistry, the pendulum is swinging back toward the recognition of physical causes as producers of mental disorders.

Drugs

Are drugs a viable answer? The National Institute for Mental Health believes so. Most of their research is directed toward controlling anxiety with increasingly sophisticated pharmaceuticals. Stronger drugs, however, have pronounced side effects, and other corrective measures *must* accompany drug therapy, or long-term treatment will be ineffective. In other words, while drugs may control excessive anxiety symptoms, they don't solve the underlying problem. And if such problems aren't dealt with, the anxiety will return and persist, creating an endless ongoing need for medication.

The Last Word

While drugs and behavioral therapy have evolved into the most utilized approaches to anxiety and fear, there is still plenty of room for improvement. Recent discoveries in the fields of neurotransmitters have opened up an entirely new approach to anxiety control using nutritional supplements (amino acids and their assistants— vitamins and minerals). This book presents a comprehensive nutritional approach to achieving such control.

2

How Nutritional Supplements Control Fears

Vitamins, minerals, and amino acids affect our emotions and even the way we think. In this chapter I will discuss the most important amino acids, vitamins, and minerals that I have used in treating serious cases of fear and anxiety and how they can change your life. The material for this chapter was gathered from medical literature, other clinicians' reports, and my own experiences. You may find it useful to refer to this chapter from time to time as you go through the book.

All of the forty or so nutrients necessary to the cell are important, but in cases of anxiety, some are more critical than others. The three vitamins most effective in controlling fear are B_1, B_3, and choline. In the mineral category, calcium is the most important. The two most essential amino acids are gamma-aminobutyric acid and glutamine. However, these elements cannot do the job alone, rather they complement and augment one another as well as others.

Thiamine, the "Moral" Vitamin

Thiamine (vitamin B_1) is a valuable nutrient for anyone who harbors excessive anxiety. Sometimes adding it to your diet is all that is necessary to eliminate a problem. However, while it diminishes some types of fears, it is only partially helpful in cases of severe anxiety. One of its main functions is to assist the cells in the breakdown of sugars and carbohydrates into glucose. Glucose together with oxygen is then converted by the body into energy. Because it provides the nervous system with energy, thiamine has a strong relationship to a healthy nervous system. I have found it to be particularly beneficial in cases of phobias and depression.

How a Deficiency of Vitamin B₁ Develops

Thiamine comes to us chiefly through whole grains such as wheat or rice. Unfortunately, a portion of each kernel is often milled away to give the grain the lighter color and finer texture that manufacturers believe the consumer wants, and vitamin B_1 usually gets lost in the process.

Because thiamine is not stored in the body, it must be supplied in the daily diet. If one eats an adequate amount of unprocessed whole grains, there is no problem. But the consumption of high-calorie and "empty" junk foods, which are nutritionally deficient, can directly cause a depletion of vitamins, especially the water-soluble B's. Nicotine, caffeine, and alcohol are also destructive to this nutrient.

After World War II, Japan experienced an epidemic of B-vitamin deficiencies. At that time, Japan had adequate food supplies, but the Japanese had fallen in love with the novelty of colas and candy brought in by Americans. Studies quickly connected B-vitamin deficiencies to the increased sugar in their diet. Laboratory research has shown that intentionally creating a B_1 deficiency is faster and easier if a large amount of sugar is consumed.

A thiamine deficiency can occur if this vitamin is overused by the hypothalamus (an area of the brain controlling neurological stability) during stress. Then biochemical enzymes start malfunctioning, and early symptoms of a B_1 deficiency begin to appear. During the initial stages, it is not uncommon for these deficiencies to cause psychological symptoms such as anxiety, irritability, fatigue, depression, and personality changes. When no other symptoms are yet apparent, such emotional changes are often dismissed as purely psychological in origin. Thiamine deficiency decreases cell energy, and a variety of symptoms may appear.

The Biochemical Lesion

It has been determined that the principal lesion takes place *in the area of cell energy metabolism*. Since the lack of energy affects all organs of the body, the number of disease symptoms can be unlimited. These differ from one person to another depending on which organs are most susceptible and may mimic or imitate a variety of diseases. (The skin lesions that are symptoms of classical beriberi develop much later.) I feel that this cellular malfunction is also a primary source of excessive fear levels and panic attacks.

Low Thiamine—High Acidity

In 1934 Peters and Thompson showed that thiamine plays a role in the metabolism of the acid pyruvate: when thiamine is deficient, there is a buildup of lactic acid in the brain, and, as we will see, lactic-acid changes in some susceptible people can precipitate panic attacks. Injections of B_1 have brought about the normalization of lactic-acid levels in the blood and brain (demonstrated by Jarvis in 1960).

Low Thiamine—Increased Sensitivity to Adrenaline

Panic patients may have an increased sensitivity to adrenaline. Because they have a preset "high sensitivity" of the nervous system, extra adrenaline will incline these patients to increased anxiety. Increased levels of adrenaline have been reported to occur in B_1-depleted animals and have also been shown to be triggers to panic attacks.

Reported Thiamine–Anxiety Connection

A 1980 study by Lonsdale and Shamberger reported that twenty patients with proven thiamine deficiencies had symptoms quite similar to those with anxiety attacks. In this group there were reports of multiple sleep disturbances, nausea, a tendency to sweat, chronic depression, dizziness, and recurring infections. Some patients exhibited unstable blood pressures, ticlike movements, neurological reflex disturbances, and abdominal and chest pains.

The Lonsdale and Shamberger study of patients with B_1 subclinical deficiencies discovered many classical signs of neurotic tension—symptoms that added up to a form of *dysautonomia* (a disturbance of the involuntary nervous system), which is the primary indicator of beriberi (thiamine deficiency). In that disease, the involuntary nervous system is affected early on and is first evidenced by unstable blood pressure, which is one of the chief symptoms of the anxiety patient.

THE INVOLUNTARY NERVOUS SYSTEM

The autonomic nervous system controls involuntary bodily functions, including glands, heart rate, blood pressure, moods, feelings, gastrointestinal activity, dilation of the eyes, and salivary flow. This system is divided into two parts which balance each other. One side, the *sympathetic nervous system*, prepares us for action—fight or flight. It speeds up our heart, raises our blood pressure, dilates our eyes, and stops gastrointestinal action. When we meet danger—either real or imagined—this part of the involuntary system takes over and gets us ready for the emergency. Adrenaline can easily launch this system into orbit.

The *parasympathetic nervous system* does just the opposite. It prepares us for rest and restoration of body needs. Our gastrointestinal system starts to digest food; our heart rate slows to normal; our muscles relax, and we feel calm. When patients become ill, whether physically or psychologically, most of the symptoms they experience are felt through the involuntary (or autonomic) nervous system.

Controlling Our Emotional System

The chief control center for the involuntary nervous system is found approximately in the center of the brain, in an area called the *hypothalamus*. The front part of the hypothalamus controls the parasympathetic nervous system; the back part controls the sympathetic nervous system.

The hypothalamus can switch our feelings and bodily functions on or off. It is vulnerable to nutritional changes and biochemical alterations just as are all other areas of the brain. When it doesn't work correctly, our entire emotional nervous system will be out of whack. Lack of adequate oxygen to the brain and body disturbs the regulation of moods and feelings. If thiamine triphosphate (a form of B_1) is depleted in the sympathetic part of the hypothalamus, there will be an increased activity in the sympathetic nervous system, and the patient will become excited and nervous. When thiamine triphosphate (B_1) is taken, the sympathetic nervous system quiets down again and the person becomes calm and relaxed, free from anxiety and tension.

Stress and the Hypothalamus

Excessive stress of any type can overload the hypothalamus. In a prolonged infection, such as mononucleosis, an extended period of grief, a serious fever, or under a heavy dose of anesthesia, the hypothalamus makes a valiant effort to maintain control; but if the impact is excessive, it can fail in its attempt. Since B_1 metabolism is important to the hypothalamus, any depletion will affect its efficiency. Thiamine metabolism in the hypothalamus may never really catch up to its needs if the deficiency is too great, or if the unlucky individual has inherited a genetic defect that causes improper reactions to stress. A normal person will eventually effect a normal resolution, but the genetically weakened person will be overwhelmed and not bounce back.

Vitamin and mineral imbalances and deficiencies that occur during times of stress are magnified if an individual uses an excessive amount of carbohydrates, nicotine, or alcohol. The stress creates a much greater need for all nutrients, especially thiamine. Since replenishment and restoration to normal balance is known to take months and even years, it is easy to see why susceptible individuals never seem to recover. They are already vulnerable, and if they have made no concentrated effort to maintain a high level of nutrition for a long period following the stress, then they may continue with borderline health. Any added stress can then endanger the precarious balance that exists. The histories of agoraphobic patients often reveal that a physical or mental trauma occurred just prior to the onset of the phobia.

Familia Dysautonomia

There is a genetic disease called familia dysautonomia with classical symptoms that might compare to those of panic patients. I am not suggesting these diseases are closely related, but in studying these patients, one can see similarities. In the case of familia dysautonomia, the cause is genetic, while in the panic patient, symptoms are possibly due to a chronic hypothalamic malfunction resulting from improper energy metabolism, which in turn has resulted from thiamine and other nutrient imbalances.

FAMILIA DYSAUTONOMIA	PANIC PATIENTS (during panic attack)
Psychological symptoms	Psychological symptoms
Neurological rash	No rash
Excessive sweating	Excessive sweating
Rapid heart	Rapid heart
Appetite changes	Unknown
Blurred vision	Vision changes
Fainting	Fainting
Fever	No fever
Headaches	Headaches at times
Breathing changes	Breathing changes
Abdominal pains	Abdominal pains
Sensitivity to cold	Cold hands
Physical Symptoms	*Physical Symptoms*
Pale	Pale
Unstable blood pressure	Unstable complaints
Distended abdomen	Abdominal complaints
Pupil changes	Dilated pupils
Tendency to infections	Some patients have an increased number of infections.
Scoliosis	No scoliosis
Sudden death	Sudden crib deaths

The chief symptomatic difference between the two groups is that panic patients have symptoms only occasionally, while the other group experiences them continuously. Both sectors, however, are genetically programmed to be susceptible. The familia dysautonomic group have symptoms from childhood, while panic-anxiety patients usually are not symptomatic until the late teens, and their illness is often preceded by separation from a significant person or a physical or mental trauma.

B_1 and Time of Recovery

Experts have found that the addition of B_1 to the diet has reversed panic symptoms and provided significant relief. The vitamin works best, however, when combined with other nutritional supplements. When restoring tissue balance in a body that has been depleted of B_1, recovery from this imbalance will be slow. No one knows why, but it is possible that the slow adaptation of the body to these depletions may have caused some compensating changes in the metabolism that are semipermanent in nature.

Thiamine Is Not the Lone Ranger

Thiamine is not a "silver bullet"—it isn't the answer to all anxieties, even though the connection between B_1 and the parts of the nervous system that produce anxiety is unquestionable. This vitamin is obviously not the sole agent responsible for anxiety disorders, and as you will see, many other nutrients play an important role.

CHOLINE

Choline, another one of the B vitamins, is primarily found in lecithin as well as in egg yolk, liver, brewer's yeast, and wheat germ. It's important to nerve transmission because it protects the health of the sheath that wraps around the nerve cells. Its other role in mental health is that it is a component of one of the most important messengers in the brain—acetylcholine. A deficiency of choline does not cause mental symptoms, but supplementary choline has a very calming effect on the body. It is useful in suppressing some anxiety and panic attack symptoms because it quiets palpitations, dizziness, balancing difficulties, and visual disturbances. It is also helpful for insomnia, hypoglycemia, and anxiety. Although choline by itself is a strong tranquilizer and could stand on its own as an aid to the anxious patient, its most beneficial effect in such instances is its potentiating effect on vitamin B_1. Without it, B_1 will not be fully effective.

Most nutritionists recommend lecithin as the chief source of choline. You can try it if you wish, but lecithin also contains large amounts of phosphorus, which can be very stimulating. Therefore, an anxious patient might take lecithin expecting some relief from nervousness, only to find that he becomes even more nervous.

BIOTIN

Biotin is a B vitamin that we seldom hear about, yet there are nutritionists who specifically recommend it for panic symptoms. Clinical experience shows that it calms anxiety, though no one knows exactly why. It may be because biotin aids in the utilization of other vitamins, such as folic acid and pantothenic acid. While there are no known toxic effects from this vitamin, lack of biotin can cause hair loss, insomnia, and a disturbed nervous system. One reason why biotin may help panic patients is that, like choline, it is essential to fat metabolism, and one function of fats is to make nerve cells healthier. A final theory is that biotin relieves panic by making vitamin B_1 work more effectively.

NIACINAMIDE

Vitamin B_3 refers to niacin or niacinamide. It is niacin that produces that sometimes irritating but harmless flush around the face and neck. Niacin is a useful aid to mental functioning and prevents allergic cravings for sugar or alcohol. It can be helpful in cases of mental illness and has been used widely in the treatment of alcoholics and psychotics. Niacinamide, on the other hand, seems to be a milder form of the vitamin and has been called nature's Valium, for it has a very powerful relaxing effect. It may be used safely in rather large doses, but beware—a few patients become depressed on niacinamide and must be switched to niacin. Niacinamide, like tryptophan, requires vitamin B_6 in order to be effective.

VITAMIN B_2 (Riboflavin)

Vitamin B_2 does not directly affect anxiety and fear, but it is supportive to the other vitamins, B_1 in particular. Riboflavin does have a positive effect on anxiety because it improves the cells' ability to utilize oxygen, and it has been found useful in combating fatigue, dizziness, trembling, and PMS symptoms. Supplementation is often necessary because it is difficult to obtain all the B_2 we need from foods. Brewer's yeast is the best source, except for those with yeast allergies.

VITAMIN B_6 (Paradoxyl-5-Phosphate)

B_6 plays a number of important roles in the body. Its most valuable function is to help the amino acids in nerve transmission. While it does not directly aid in controlling anxiety and fear, it is extremely supportive to those amino acids and vitamins that do, particularly niacinamide. It's also critical to mineral balance and normal functioning of nervous tissue. Without B_6, there may be a greater tendency toward hypoglycemia, which is one of the triggers to panic attacks. A lack of B_6 can cause muscle weakness, nervousness, irritability, tingling hands, and depression. It has been found helpful in treating PMS, epilepsy, insomnia, mental illness, headaches, stress, alcoholism, and other problems related to high anxiety levels.

FOLIC ACID

In overcoming anxiety and fear, folic acid plays a role as a coenzyme or helper to the other vitamins and minerals. It is also important because it helps stabilize the hormone system and is particularly beneficial to female sex hormone normality. Sex hormone imbalances are one of the triggers to panic attacks. Folic acid has been used in the treatment of alcoholism, mental illness, stress, and fatigue, and I have found it very useful in dealing with PMS.

PANTOTHENIC ACID

This vitamin is a helpmate to vitamin B_1 and to the adrenal gland, which makes it useful in fighting panic and phobias. It is also necessary for the formation of sex hormones. Pantothenic acid can benefit those with hypoglycemia, stress, fatigue, depression, alcoholism, abdominal pain, headaches, epilepsy, fainting, insomnia, and various forms of mental illness. PA also decreases lactic acid buildup by helping the body eliminate it more rapidly.

COD LIVER OIL (Essential Fatty Acids)

Vitamin F found in cod liver oil is a mixture of unsaturated oils. While it does not directly affect anxiety and fear, it is very necessary for its impact on calcium. It is also necessary for good oxygenation of tissues and for normal glandular functioning. It has been found helpful in cases of PMS, alcoholism, mental illness, dizziness, and fatigue.

Balancing Vitamins

As you can see, I have left out a number of vitamins, but not because they aren't important. In Chapter 4, I have recommended the best all-around multivitamin I have been able to find. When you use individual vitamins for some particular clinical effect, it's essential that you take a good multivitamin along with the specific vitamins in order to keep other deficiencies from developing. I also believe that periodically one should stop all nutritional supplements for a week or so to let the body rebalance itself. As we artificially treat ourselves, we want to be sure we allow our body some control over its own balance in other areas of metabolism.

CALCIUM AND ANXIETY HAVE BEEN TOGETHER FOR A LONG TIME

For more than forty years, family doctors have given anxious and disturbed patients calcium by intravenous injection. Doctors noticed its calming effect many years ago and suggested a bedtime glass of milk to induce sleep. Early on, nutritionists and nutritional authors wrote about the value of calcium in producing relaxation, which, defined simply, means the removal of anxiety.

My Early Experiences with Calcium

Some years ago, when I first started to use nutritional supplements in the treatment of psychological problems, a young lady asked me for help during an early stage of social phobia. She realized that she was beginning to develop an aversion to crowds and wanted to deal with the problem before it completely controlled her.

She explained her problem to me: "When I go into a dental office where a group of people are waiting, I become uneasy. Sometimes I have to walk out into the hall to wait my turn. I tell the nurse I need some fresh air and ask her to call me when the dentist is ready. Larger crowds like those at an amusement park completely overwhelm me. Any group of people tightly packed together makes me feel panicky."

I asked this patient, on a trial basis, to take some calcium tablets before she went to crowded locations. Later she reported a surprising lack of fear or anxiety even in the midst of a "mob" at Disneyland. This was a very simple phobia, of course, but it still shows that the biochemical approach to psychological disorders can work quickly and effectively. At about this same time, I read a report, "Lactate in Anxiety" by Pitts and McClure, in the *New England Journal of Medicine*, 1967, which stated that an excess of lactic acid might be the cause of some types of anxiety, and that calcium might alleviate its buildup.

I tried calcium lactate tablets on another patient who had a fear of flying. She took four tablets while she was waiting to board her plane and reported that she suffered no fears at all during takeoff or while in flight. Again, this was a very mild phobia, but it proved a point. Critics may say, of course, that the calcium merely provided a placebo effect, but I don't agree. These two patients used this technique successfully time after time, over a period of months and eventually years. Placebo effects generally wear off usually after about ninety days.

A Common Ailment—Minor
Calcium Imbalances

The body will develop symptoms if it is deficient in calcium, or if the calcium is just not properly placed. One of the earliest and most common signals of a calcium problem is tingling in the toes and fingers (both sides of the body at the same time), and around the mouth and lips. It is often mistakenly diagnosed as poor circulation. Muscle cramping and low blood pressure are two other early symptoms of calcium deficiency. Many women report experiencing these symptoms occasionally but are unaware of what causes them.

It's Easy to Create an Imbalance
in Calcium Metabolism

During the last fifteen years there have sprung up a number of intense, personal interaction groups such as EST and Life-Spring. As part of their processes, these groups inflict intense psychological pressures on their members in order to create not only intellectual but also highly emotional experiences.

   While undergoing the emotional outbursts that frequently occur, some individuals suddenly start to experience a tightening in their arms and fingers. The fingers straighten, spread, and then "lock up." The hands and arms start to bow toward the midline of the body. When this happens, they are said to be "crabbing" because the posture of their arms begins to mimic a crab's claws. In classical medicine, this is called Chvostek's sign and is caused by a deficiency of available calcium. In these impact groups, "crabbing" is not caused by a real calcium deficiency, but rather a relative deficiency due to a shift in calcium resulting from an intense emotional reaction adversely affecting the lungs and breathing patterns.

   Calcium levels in the blood can also be changed by the thyroid, parathyroid, and gonadal glands. They can also be changed by alterations in breathing patterns, vitamin D, acidity or alkalinity levels, and the levels of essential fatty acids.

Calcium Works—Even in the Lab

As already mentioned, even in the laboratory calcium has been successful in alleviating anxiety and panic attacks. Although this has not been uniformly true in all cases, it has worked for many. With a number of patients, I have found calcium, along with other nutrients, to be very helpful in mild to moderate cases of phobia and panic. It has not been as helpful as I would have liked, however, for the agoraphobic, although it is of some benefit to these patients.

Calcium—The Key Element

Because the body cannot function without the major minerals, it is difficult to say which mineral (sodium, potassium, calcium, or magnesium) is the most important. They all hold key positions. On balance, however, calcium seems to be a shade ahead of the others. This is primarily because calcium controls the effects of the other major minerals and the amino acids.

- Calcium controls the porelike openings that connect the inside of the cells to the outside.
- Calcium controls the biogenic amino chemicals that pass messages between nerve cells.
- Calcium is the structural skeleton of the cell.
- Calcium carries messages throughout the interior of the cells.
- Calcium plays a key role in cell energy.

Calcium Holds the Key
to Stable Nerves

Human cells might be described as soap bubbles grouped together. They are not, however, empty bubbles. Rather, they are bulging with an active and constantly moving substance called protoplasm. A thousand human cells placed in a row reach only the length of one inch. The entire body is a collection of trillions of tiny cells. Even though they are tightly packed together, some space still exists between them, which is filled with a nutrient-rich fluid. Some of these tiny cells are specialists and others aren't. Most specialist cells, such as muscle or nerve cells, can be activated, and once in motion, they perform a specific duty. For example, a nerve cell may carry a message to a muscle cell that contracts and causes an arm or a leg to move.

Many of these effects are orchestrated by calcium. For example, when a nerve cell is being turned on (activated), an electrical current moves down the nerve. Minerals located outside the cell rush to the inside, and, vice versa, minerals inside the cell rush to get outside. These minerals cannot just penetrate the cell wall; instead, they must pass through special tunnels or channels. These channels can be opened or closed, and like gates, most of them are controlled by the gatekeeper, calcium.

Without Calcium, Nothing Happens

An experiment was conducted in which a frog's heart was set, still beating, into a bowl of fluid containing all the necessary nutrients to keep it alive, except calcium. The heart quickly stopped beating. It was proof that without calcium, all nerve impulses in the heart as well as the body slow down or come to a halt.

We now get some idea of how powerful calcium balance is to our nerves—they simply can't function without it. And there's more. Nerve cells do not stretch from our brain to our toes. They link together like long pieces of string placed end to end, with a small space between the end of one nerve and the beginning of another. When an electrical impulse is traveling along, it eventually stops at the end of the nerve. How, then, does the activated nerve signal the tip of the next nerve to pass the message on? The first nerve does so by releasing a chemical messenger from its tip which crosses the gap and activates the tip of the next nerve. This chemical messenger sent across the gap is released by our old friend, calcium.

Calcium—The Rock

Without bones, your body would be nothing more than a blob of tissue as wobbly as Jell-O. This same need for structure also exists in each individual cell, and that structure, too, is provided by calcium. It is important to note that arachidonic acid (a fat) and the other essential fatty acids are helpers that assist calcium in strengthening and regulating the cells, as well as other biochemical functions. Their absence is the reason why there are times when calcium fails to produce the expected results. In such cases, these essential fatty acids must be supplied in conjunction with the calcium. I have often seen dramatic improvement in symptoms when these elements are added in proper amounts to the calcium intake. Like most nutritional supplements, essential fatty acids are easily obtainable at any health food store.

Calcium—The Messenger Inside the Cell

In the role of gatekeeper, calcium has the important function of allowing water and nutrients to pass through the tunnels in the cell walls to the inside. Inside the cell, calcium has another busy schedule. Functioning as a messenger, it helps regulate many of the cell's most fundamental processes, such as movement, muscle contraction, cell fertilization and pregnancy, the growth of the cell (calcium regulates DNA synthesis), hormone functions, movements of other minerals, and even cell death. (Most cells are constantly being replaced.)

In between the cells, calcium also plays a role associated with blood clotting and controlling communication between non-nerve cells.

Calcium and Energy

For our purposes here, we are interested in knowing how calcium can help us preserve our mental health, or in some cases, regain it. We have just discussed why calcium is so vital to the workings of our nerves and the chemical functions of our cells. These things of course affect our mental health, but the two most important functions of calcium are its direct impact inside the nerve cells and its role in helping each cell produce energy.

Mitochondria are small subunit packs in the cell. They create the energy that helps everything run smoothly, but their job is compromised when there is a lack of available calcium. This deficiency inside the mitochondria prevents the conversion of oxygen to energy. A buildup of lactic acid results which can reach levels which trigger panic attacks in susceptible individuals. Since calcium and oxygen are both necessary for energy buildup, a lack of oxygen will have the same effect as a lack of calcium—it triggers panic in certain people.

Still Another Function of Calcium

With so many important functions, it's easy to see why a sufficiency of calcium is so vital. In addition, calcium is a powerful alkalizer. Since acidity at the local level in the cells causes the lack of oxygen that sets off panic, an alkalizer may neutralize the acidity and allow more cell oxygenation. While it is alkalizing, the extra calcium is now available to perform its various other important functions.

Calcium and Mood

Calcium has been strongly implicated in mood disorders. Very slight changes in calcium blood levels and shifts in its location in the brain can lead to anything from euphoria to irritability and anxiety. Although the lowering of calcium levels has been effective in the treatment of manic depression, this is contradictory to my experience with panic and fear patients, and I have no good explanation for why this occurs. Knowing the importance of biochemical individuality, I am always conscious of any positive or negative effects of vitamins, and I make changes accordingly. Overall, I have found that calcium helps control anxiety.

Other Minerals

A multimineral tablet is generally helpful to anxiety patients and is necessary for anxiety control. Except for calcium, however, I have not found any other single mineral particularly helpful. Some literature suggests that magnesium has tranquilizing properties, but I have seen it produce just the opposite reaction if given in too high doses. Because of this, I have limited my recommendations to small amounts, perhaps 50 to 100 mg three times a day, as a support to other vitamins or amino acids. Sodium (salt) is useful for hypoglycemic nervous tension or headaches, so it could also be helpful in blocking hypoglycemia as a trigger to panic attacks.

AMINO ACIDS

There are two major reasons why we want to focus your attention on amino acids. We can see by lab tests changes in the levels of certain amino acids in the plasma and urine which seem to be associated with various physical and mental disorders. When these amino-acid levels are brought, by supplementation, into proper balance, symptoms are reduced or disappear. Certain amino acids, when sufficiently supplemented, will travel to the brain where they are made into, or function as, neurohormones. These neurohormones help improve nerve transmission and relieve symptoms such as depression and moodiness.

What Are Amino Acids?

Amino acids are small molecules that, when "strung together," make up proteins. There are twenty-two amino acids in the circulating blood, and they are the main source of nitrogen in the body. Proteins form most of the tissue in the body, except fatty tissue. After digestion, amino acids are absorbed, and most are sent to the liver or kidneys, while those involved in muscle contractions go directly to the muscles. Still others form connective tissues, brain, skin, bone matrix, and other body systems. Hormones, antibodies, blood elements, and enzymes are all proteins. There are at least 1,600 basic proteins in the human body.

Amino acids can be made into hormones and various components of our immune system. They regulate nerve excitation as well as acid base and water balance, and they are a necessary part of the enzymes. Along with vitamins and minerals, enzymes control all biochemical reactions in the body.

Amino acids are the building blocks of life. Of the twenty-two amino acids, the body manufactures only fourteen. The others must be supplied through diet. These "essential amino acids" are found in meat, fish, poultry, and dairy products.

Dietary habits influence the level of amino acids in the body. For example, vegetables are low in lysine, so vegetarians may develop a deficiency of lysine. Diseases can also greatly alter the amounts available for metabolic processes, even with a completely adequate diet. Deficiencies such as these should be made up by the intake of supplemental amino acids. It is important that all twenty-two amino acids be taken along with any individual ones specifically indicated in a supplement program.

Amino Acids Need Vitamins and Minerals

All chemical reactions involved in metabolic processes require the presence of other substances for the reactions to proceed normally. Such substances are called coenzymes. Vitamins and minerals are coenzymes in amino acid metabolism. Amino acids don't work without them. In fact, each individual reaction of an enzyme requires two helpers (coenzymes), a specific vitamin, and a specific mineral.

Analysis of Amino Acids

Plasma and urine analysis for amino-acid levels has been available for twenty-five years. Until recently, this test has been used only in research science, with no real clinical application. Over the years, however, physicians have begun to recognize distinct patterns in these analyses that accompany specific physical and psychological disorders. At the same time, Dr. Richard Wurtman and other researchers have discovered that amino acid levels in our diets are directly connected to our mental and physical health. Gradually, correlations between lab analysis and illness have been developed.

Amino-acid-analysis testing is made available through Aatron Medical Services, a division of Tyson and Associates in Santa Monica, California. Aatron's laboratory performs a complete analysis of all amino acids and metabolites found in plasma and urine. This test is an excellent guide to proper supplementation since, in essence, it "fingerprints" each patient's deficiencies, so that an individualized program can be designed from test results and consideration of the patient's other symptoms.

Should a patient already be taking medication, it may be gradually eliminated in favor of the amino-acid supplementation. It takes time for any nutritional or metabolic therapy to correct chronic disorders. However, the success rate of amino-acid therapy is quite good—especially when the patient follows a program of sound nutrition and avoids chemicals or foods to which he or she is allergic.

Which patients have done well on amino-acid therapy? Those suffering from unexplained fatigue or stress, where other common treatments have been unhelpful, patients with all types of depression (including psychotic depression), some cases of schizophrenia, hyperactivity in children, aggressive or destructive behavior in children, learning disorders, mood swings in adults, some phobias, anxiety, and manic depression.

Amino Acids and Mental Illness

Let's examine the connection between psychological disorders and amino acid imbalance. Researchers are now able to differentiate between depression and anxiety in linking these disorders to patterns found in amino acid analysis. Absolute certainty is not *always* possible, but the patterns are distinct enough to help assist in the diagnoses of many cases.

For example, gamma-aminobutyric acid is usually not found in appreciable amounts in the urine of normal adults. However, extremely high amounts of this amino acid are found in those suffering from agoraphobia and other neurotic anxieties. As you will see later, gamma-aminobutyric acid is a neurohormone in the brain which serves to calm anxiety. The presence of excessive amounts of this amino acid in the urine tells us that the body is desperately trying to calm down anxiety by producing huge amounts of it. But something is wrong. It is all being eliminated in the urine and is not being utilized by the body. Perhaps a defective mechanism or receptor is preventing the amino acid from being properly utilized. Whatever the reason, we have a marker for anxiety.

In another example, a normal plasma–amino-acid analysis test will show a two-to-one ratio between tyrosine and tryptophan. Often when the ratio drops to one-to-one, symptoms of depression are present. Analysis of amino-acid levels in this way provides us with a "window" to the biochemical interactions in the body.

Treating Anxiety with Messenger Amino Acids

There are three steps required in proper amino-acid supplementation. First, we must determine just what the deficiencies are. This is done by analyzing the plasma and urine through a process called Amino Acid Ion Exchange Chromatography (or the Aatron Medical Service Test). Second, the findings of the chromatography test are interpreted in conjunction with the patient's history and symptoms. Third, a program of supplementation is instituted, tailored to the individual patient.

For very mild cases of anxiety, we may, without doing lab tests, simply use those amino acids previous experience has shown to be effective in treating certain disorders. For example, L-tyrosine and L-tryptophan have been useful in treating cases of depression because they are converted by the body into neuroactive agents necessary for synaptic transmission: neurotransmitters, neuromodulators, and neurohormones.

Both techniques (using clinical experience or laboratory analysis as a guide) are effective. Both are backed by years of clinical experiments. The difference lies in the procedure. The amino acid analysis test must be obtained with the help of a physician. The second technique of simply adding to the diet specific amino acids, selected on the basis of symptoms, may be tried first, although a physician's guidance is always recommended.

An Amino Acid Useful in the Treatment of Anxiety

GLUTAMINE

This amino acid helps in the treatment of phobias, anxiety, and panic by producing energy without causing nervousness. It also makes the mind more alert without causing one to feel "wired" or "hyper." It accomplishes this partially through its ability to detoxify the ammonia buildup in cells. Another way it contributes to a sense of well-being and energy is that as it passes through the kidneys, it helps the body retain both potassium and sodium.

Glutamine is beneficial to patients undergoing stress. Stress usually begins by creating vague feelings of discomfort; then as it worsens, it starts to produce functional disease, at which point it becomes a primarily biochemical disturbance. If stress continues long enough and severely enough, the body tissues begin to degenerate, and the first place the tissues start to break down is in the stomach. This vital organ must manufacture a million new cells each hour in order to resist the effect of acid strong enough to burn its way through metal; therefore, when the body weakens ever so slightly, this acid starts to break through and produce painful symptoms. That is why people under severe stress so often develop ulcers. Glutamine promotes the regeneration of the linings of the digestive tract and, as such, can be labeled an antistress nutrient.

It also helps control cravings for such items as sugar and alcohol and is therefore useful in preventing the excessive intake of two of the major triggers to panic attacks.

Its most profound effect is in stimulating clearer thinking. It has been useful in improving brain functions of patients with mental retardation and epilepsy, at the same time improving memory and, surprisingly, enhancing physical dexterity.

I have never seen glutamine produce toxic effects in any of my patients. I have therefore prescribed fairly high amounts for many months with no apparent side effects. I suggest that my patients take four to six tablets or more as often as needed, but no more frequently than every four hours. Most of my patients don't use it on a regular basis, but only as needed.

GABA (Gamma-Aminobutyric Acid)

GABA is not a constituent of proteins; instead, it is made from glutamic acid in the nervous system. This amino acid is critically essential for brain metabolism because it functions as a regulator of neuronal activity. It produces calmness and tranquility by inhibiting the excessive firing of nerve cells that are keeping the mind overactive. Another way in which it can have a tranquilizing effect on the body is by making vitamin B_3 (niacinamide) bind more closely to its docking site on the cells. GABA, when given to lab animals, prevents the development of learned helplessness. GABA has been a major calming agent in many of my patients.

TRYPTOPHAN

Tryptophan is an essential amino acid, which means it cannot be manufactured by the body and must be obtained through the diet. Certain nutrients make it work more effectively. For example, if zinc is taken along with tryptophan, it will produce better results. Fruit, fruit juice, or some other rapid form of carbohydrates will maximize the uptake of tryptophan for a calming effect. Vitamin B_6 is also a vital helpmate (coenzyme). If there is a deficiency in the body of B_6, there will be a failure in the normal metabolism of tryptophan, and a toxic, abnormal metabolite called xanthurenic acid is formed. Too much xanthurenic acid can cause diabetes. This amino acid has a reputation for being a good tranquilizer, however, and has often been used to treat insomnia.

There are several ways in which tryptophan calms the nervous system. First of all, it is a necessary building block for serotonin. Serotonin is a brain neurohormone which, when not present in excess, has a relaxing effect on the mind. Second, tryptophan is converted into nicotinic acid, a nutrient essential throughout the brain. Assisting in good normal metabolism, nicotinic acid has a settling effect also.

Patients with mental disorders often complain of insomnia or poor-quality sleep. This disturbance in natural body rhythm adds more stress to an already overstressed body. Getting a good night's sleep is always one of the first places to start in restoring normality to a frazzled system.

Tryptophan has often been touted as a good "sleeping pill." If you have only a mild problem with insomnia, you may find it quite useful; however, if your problem is more severe, you will probably be disappointed, for it usually induces sleep but doesn't maintain it. Consult Chapter 14 for additional remedies to sleep disturbances.

Tryptophan has also been used in the treatment of anxiety, either by itself or in conjunction with medications. My experience is that while it may help some patients, it is of limited value for the majority. In some cases it may even have an adverse effect. Some patients report they are not clearheaded or simply "don't feel well," so use caution. Most health food stores carry the product and it usually comes in 500 mg tablets.

For anxiety I start my patients with one 500 mg tablet every four hours throughout the day and again at bedtime. I increase the dose gradually if I start to see results. But I emphasize that although tryptophan is a nutrient, when it is used as a drug, it may have side effects—often in the form of drowsiness—and like any sedative, should not be taken when driving or operating machinery.

Paradoxically, tryptophan has also been used for depression, and with some success. In a British study (Picknold) the antidepressant clomipramine was paired with L-tryptophan, one gram, three times daily, up to two grams, four times daily, and was successful in relieving depression.

Clomipramine's main function is to inhibit the re-uptake of serotonin in the brain. This means that more serotonin remains in the brain to combat depression. Tryptophan helps by transforming into serotonin when it reaches the brain through the blood. Thus it creates additional serotonin to potentiate the drug clomipramine. Test results indicate that tryptophan has no effect on agoraphobia or social phobias.

PHENYLALANINE

This is an essential amino acid. In the body it is converted to another amino acid called tyrosine. When it is combined with aspartic acid, it becomes the sweetener aspartame, and has long been used as a tonic because it is a stimulant to the energy system. As phenylalanine is processed in the body, it produces adrenaline which in turn provides energy.

This amino acid is useful in some types of depression, especially in cases of premenstrual syndrome. I advise my patients to take one tablet every time they feel depressed, up to two tablets at a time. In some patients it has produced results within five minutes. But again, caution is advised. Too much phenylalanine can cause irritability, anger, and nervousness.

One patient describes her experience: "I was crying for no reason. First I would get angry and lash out at people, then I would start to feel sorry for myself. I had no control over my emotions. But the minute I put the tablet under my tongue, I felt myself getting better. It was like a miracle."

Sometimes I tell patients to crush a tablet and keep it under their tongue for a few minutes because this method produces a very rapid response.

Phenylalanine should not be used for anxiety because it only makes the patient more tense and nervous, but it can be effective for patients with hypoglycemia and low blood pressure. Seldom do these two diseases exist separately, so I will discuss them as one. Phenylalanine produces adrenaline, and adrenaline is the primary hormone used by the body to raise blood pressure. Adrenaline also opposes insulin and assists the body in the release of stored sugar. The availability of this sugar to the cells of the body and a higher blood pressure mean the end of hypoglycemia symptoms.

Placebo Effect—Is That All It Is?

A placebo is an inert substance given to patients in hopes of improving their condition. It relies totally on the user's belief in its efficiency. In other words, "It will work if the patient *thinks* it will."

Do vitamins ever fall into this category? Some readers would love to jump to this conclusion. There are, however, good answers to those critics. First of all, placebo effects are generally not long lasting; at most they "work" for about ninety days, then the benefits decline as reality sets in. Many nutritionists, however, have seen the beneficial effects of nutritional supplements last for years, which clearly rules out any placebo effect.

It can also be argued that all forms of psychotherapy, if they work, are nothing more than a sort of placebo. Positive expectations are part and parcel of any therapy, whether it be drug, vitamin, or psychotherapy. If there is some placebo effect to nutritional therapy, it is no greater than that which exists in any other form of treatment.

Summary

I have explained how each individual nutrient calms anxiety. By itself, no one nutrient is sufficient to do the job. Skillfully combined they become a symphony. Other nutritional supplements must also be used with them for further fine-tuning. The formulas found in the chapters to follow represent years of experience with thousands of patients. They have worked for me and my patients; they will work for you.

CAUTION: Individual amino acids, used in large doses for long periods of time, may produce toxic effects. There are, however, several rules of safety that will protect you. First: don't exceed 1500 mg a day. Larger amounts should be taken only under the supervision of a physician or a nutritionist. Second: when taking individual amino acids, always take daily at least 1000 mg of a full-spectrum amino acid tablet or capsule (19 to 22 amino acids). Shortages of other amino acids are thus avoided. Third: while using individual amino acid therapy, always include at least 150 mg of B_6 daily. Studies have suggested that most of the toxic effects created by taking large amounts of amino acids are caused by insufficient B_6. B_6 is necessary to accomplish the full metabolism of the amino acids.

3

Triggers, Environmental Initiators of Fears

Many patients and doctors do not recognize the subtle, invisible stressors that can arouse fear and panic. These terrible feelings occur because of a disorganized and disturbed nervous system. It's preset to go off like an explosion in situations where a more normal nervous system would react far less dramatically. What often provokes this overreaction is a "trigger," the sight or sound or thought of a feared object or situation.

There are, however, other kinds of triggers that physically destabilize the nervous system. In these cases the frightened individual is fully aware of the object or situation that provokes the fear and panic but is often unaware of other less obvious contributors to the attack. The purpose of this chapter is to identify those physiological triggers so that they can be avoided or controlled.

Triggers (Inciters, Exciters, Tormentors, Instigators, Provokers)

An inciter or trigger is the switch that "turns on," "starts up," or at least intensifies a particular reaction. Here we will cover a multitude of conditions that activate the switch that escalates us into fear and anxiety.

Why is it necessary to understand the function of triggers? The answer is obvious. If you know where a reaction originates, you have a chance to stop the cycle in its first stages, and you also have the advantage of knowing points along the way where you can intervene and block panic from progressing further.

This is a list of the most common triggers. I will explain each one, how it causes the panic switch to activate, and what you can do to intervene or prevent it.

1. Processed sugar or excess natural carbohydrates
2. Caffeine
3. Alcohol
4. Drugs
5. Exercise
6. Hormone imbalance
7. Lights
8. Heat
9. Physical illness
10. Sudden shock and emotions
11. Environmental chemicals
12. Foods

Trigger No. 1—Processed Sugar

Sugar is a well-known antinutrient. Because it contains no vitamins within its structure, it must draw upon the body's store of vitamins in order to be properly metabolized. In an already depleted individual, sugar can serve as a trigger to panic. It is also notorious for causing hypoglycemia, another precipitator of increased lactic-acid and decreased calcium levels, both known to provoke panic attacks. (See Chapter 2.) It should be noted that excessive amounts of natural carbohydrates, such as honey or fruits, may also cause the same types of biochemical changes in susceptible individuals. I have had patients whose panic attacks were activated by fruits such as oranges; eliminating this single trigger decreased the number of panic attacks they had.

Trigger No. 2—Caffeine

Caffeine is another effective inducer of panic attacks. In one lab experiment, caffeine administered in doses equivalent to five cups of coffee produced panic attacks in half the susceptible patients. Even in normal subjects, eight cups of coffee, when ingested rapidly, can produce symptoms similar to a panic attack. One possible reason is caffeine's antithiamine effect. It destroys vitamin B_1 and may also affect calcium balance. Caffeine is thought to produce its activating effects by blocking receptors in the brain which receive *adenosine*, a brain chemical which is a naturally occurring sedative. Caffeine also produces anxiety through the benzodiazepine system, and stimulates an adrenaline response. It is clear that there are many ways caffeine can bring on fear and panic.

Trigger No. 3—Alcohol

Some may think it strange that alcohol, which is a depressant, can trigger panic attacks, especially when it is commonly used by many as a way of combating tension and anxiety. Dr. Westol, the German physician who in the late 1800s was the first to label anxiety attacks "agoraphobia," in fact prescribed alcohol for his patients.

Although alcohol initially suppresses anxiety symptoms, it is metabolized as a simple carbohydrate (sugar), and it reacts in the body in the same way as any other sugar. Most notably, it depletes the body of its stores of vitamins and minerals. Nearly everyone is aware that delirium tremens and cirrhosis of the liver are direct results of vitamin and mineral deficiencies caused by excessive use of alcohol, and that these conditions can occur when the body is not supplied with adequate amounts of nutritious foods.

Alcohol, when it goes full cycle, intensifies the very problem it may have been intended to relieve, by setting up a chain reaction that triggers panic attacks. The patient experiences relief from panic after a shot of alcohol, then finds that as it wears off, his anxiety returns more intensely than before, creating a treacherous and hard-to-break cycle.

Trigger No. 4—Drugs

Both legal and recreational drugs are known to deplete the body of vitamins and minerals. Usually the body can make the necessary adjustments, unless usage is chronic. Ten days on an antibiotic, for example, is not going to produce a noticeable effect on the body's nutrition, but long-term use of medications such as birth control pills, tranquilizers, antihistamines, and antiarthritics can gradually rob the body of significant amounts of vitamins to a point where symptoms develop.

Theophylline, for example, is a drug found in chocolate, coffee, and other common foods and beverages. Its stimulatory effects are well known, and it has often been implicated in panic attacks. It's been well documented that birth control pills produce a vitamin B_6 deficiency, along with the loss of other nutrients. Such chronic imbalances have definite effects on the body's acid-base balances and many of the body's enzyme systems. In susceptible individuals, drugs, like alcohol, which initially prevent anxiety may, over the long term, create conditions which perpetuate anxiety and leave the person even more drug dependent. (See page 90 for a discussion of the dangers of drugs in the treatment of panic.) As with alcohol, withdrawal from marijuana or cocaine may cause panic attacks along with other symptoms. Recreational drugs cause significant depletion of nutritional stores, and I have seen panic and phobic symptoms worsen quickly with their use, causing some patients to become almost psychotic. They severely intensify symptoms of PMS.

Trigger No. 5—Exercise

Physical exertion is known to produce a sharp rise in lactic acid, up to twenty times the normal level in average persons, and many times higher in susceptible individuals. Exercise can therefore be a potent trigger to panic attacks. Circumstances vary, of course, according to the individual. Many panic patients do not experience attacks after exercise and may even find it beneficial in combating anxiety.

Trigger No. 6—Hormone Imbalance

Changes in sex hormone levels in the blood can sometimes trigger panic attacks. In one study (Leibowitz and Kelin 1981), panic attacks occurred in three women within a year of surgical removal of their ovaries. Three other patients reported that panic symptoms began shortly after their uteruses were removed. Another three patients suffered panic attacks within the month following childbirth, and two others complained of these symptoms one week prior to delivery.

A patient of mine started having panic attacks shortly after she was placed on birth control pills by another physician. When she suspected a relationship, she discontinued the pills, but the panic attacks persisted, and it was at that point that she contacted me for treatment. Happily, her condition was easily controlled with nutritional supplements.

Anxiety attacks that often begin or worsen during the premenstrual period may be linked to excess progesterone, which has been found to precipitate such attacks in laboratory experiments. Researchers assume there is an excess of progesterone during the premenstrual time. In men, the opposite effect occurs—progesterone tends to have a calming effect. (In a disease called primary central hypoventilation, largely a male disorder, progesterone supplementation has been extremely effective.)

There are important changes in the acid–alkaline blood balance during the second half of the menstrual cycle. One important cause of this is the level of progesterone. High or low levels may set up conditions for panic. If we know this we can control progesterone and therefore control panic.

I have successfully treated hundreds of patients for PMS, and I believe that I have some valuable observations on this condition. I have noticed that an extremely high percentage of these patients experience panic attacks only while suffering from PMS and not at other times of the month. Of course agoraphobic and phobic patients may have anxiety attacks anytime, but these tend to occur more frequently during the premenstrual phase.

In milder cases, I have seen complete remission of panic attacks in all patients when the PMS symptoms have been corrected by using progesterone in very small amounts. It is paradoxical that although administration of excessive amounts of progesterone is known to cause panic attacks, patients with PMS, a disorder supposedly caused by a deficiency or dysfunction of progesterone, often experience increasingly frequent panic attacks; but when progesterone is given, the panic attacks completely cease. Why this occurs, I am not sure. I know only that a few hundred women will bear witness to this fact; perhaps, like so many mysteries of medicine, what works in one patient may not work in another.

Other hormones are known to have an effect on fear. An overactive thyroid, for example, is known to cause the development of an increased number of beta-adrenergic receptors in various tissues in both animals and humans. (See Chapter 17.) This increase causes the individual to become hypersensitive to any form of stimulation, physical or mental, and may result in anxiety and panic.

Trigger No. 7—Lights

The effect of lights on *chemically sensitive patients* is well known. It is suspected that lighting may also have some effect on *panic syndrome patients*. There is a difference between incandescent lights, which produce a continuous spectrum of all visible wavelengths, and fluorescent lighting, which contains occasional spiked line radiation. A number of agoraphobics experience sensitivity to fluorescent lighting and report aggravated symptoms in its presence.

Light visible to humans measures between 350 and 750 nanometers. Light is transmitted to the retina, to the optic nerve tract, through the lateral geniculate body, to the optic radiations, and finally to the occipital cortex. But not *all* fibers from the retina take this route. Some go to an area where they help control visual reflexes (i.e., pupillary size). Another more newly discovered path, called the *retinal hypothalamic path*, reaches from the retina to the suprachiasmatic nuclei of the hypothalamus. This is vitally important because it relates to the setting of biological clocks. The range of light frequencies to which this pathway is sensitive is not known, but it has been well demonstrated that human and animal menstrual cycles, for example, are greatly influenced by light exposure.

The problem with fluorescent lights is that they flicker. These low-pressure mercury lamps emit 90 percent of their energy at a wavelength of 253.7 nm. This is near the ultraviolet range, but there are smaller peaks in the visible range. Problems arise from the alternating current from which they are powered. The lamp discharges on both the positive and negative cycles, causing it to flicker at about 120 Hz. The coating on the inside of the glass tube is supposed to receive these impulses and emit a continuous glow. This so-called smooth light is not completely masked, and when most people look steadily at a fluorescent lamp, they can see at least a slight flicker. As the lamp ages, the two phases of the alternating current discharge unequally, and the flickering increases.

In my office I frequently hear certain agoraphobics complain they are bothered by the lighting in markets or malls. Some are so sensitive they cannot even enter these areas. Others become more and more uneasy or anxious and are eventually forced to leave. Allergists and clinical ecologists often report seeing these patients develop more tolerance to fluorescent lights as their sensitivities to environmental chemicals, pollens, and foods decline.

Trigger No. 8—Heat

I know of no actual studies involving the relationship between anxiety and heat; but in the Palm Springs area, where the temperature sometimes exceeds 115 degrees, the local psychologists tell me that they often have long waiting lists of patients during the hottest months, and that their practice falls off during the cooler months. In their opinion, heat *does* increase anxiety levels.

Trigger No. 9—Physical Illness

Although a physical illness usually does not cause panic per se, it may still set the stage. In Chapter 17 I have listed cases in which anxiety developed after general surgery or following viral infections. For example, in one case a female requested treatment for fatigue, depression, and panic attacks and was found to be severely anemic. All of her symptoms disappeared when her anemia was successfully treated.

Trigger No. 10—Sudden Shock and Emotions

Case histories indicate that sudden surprises may cause the onset of fright and panic attacks. Overresponders to surprise don't seem to be able to readjust gradually. It is common knowledge that strong emotions may also create the internal chaos that predisposes some patients to anxiety attacks.

Trigger No. 11—Environmental Chemicals

Allergic reactions are probably the most frequently unrecognized cause of illness in the United States. The three major sources of allergies are pollens, foods, and chemicals. Our focus at the moment will be on chemical sensitivities. No one would question the concept that our bodies can tolerate only a limited amount of contamination before illness develops. But what actually produces the illness? Is it allergy, toxicity (enzyme blockage), free radical tissue damage, hypoxia (lack of oxygen to tissues), or some other mechanism? The answer may lie in a combination of factors, but at this time, our knowledge is limited. We do know, however, that some patients are exquisitely sensitive to micro amounts of chemicals, and that these individuals will react when exposed to even tiny particles of offending substances.

Modern chemical hazards include caffeine, nicotine, alcohol, salicylates, formaldehyde, phenols, pesticides, fumigants, herbicides, plasticizers, fertilizers, food additives, fuels, household chemicals (soaps, solvents, cleaners, etc.), both prescription and illegal drugs, cosmetics (perfumes, after-shave lotions, etc.), and yes, even drinking water. There are enough chemicals in tap water to make some chemically sensitive patients significantly ill. At the present time there are more than 60,000 chemicals in current use.

All of these substances can easily penetrate the body through the skin, lungs, or gastrointestinal tract. Once invaded, the body will try to detoxify itself as quickly as possible, before it suffers damage. If the immune system is strong enough, the body's own mechanisms may be sufficient. However, much of the time, chemicals are not destroyed by the body, and they simply get locked into such areas as connective tissue, and especially fat tissue. From these locations, they may slowly leach back into the system and produce a slow form of poisoning.

Occupational medicine has long accepted the fact that long-term chemical exposure may cause any number of diseases, including malignancies. Ever more frequently, Western man is experiencing excessive loads on basic body defenses. This weakening of our immune system often leads to food and chemical hypersensitivities and produces symptoms of both psychological and physical disease. Since these sensitivities can trigger forms of mental illness, it's certainly logical that they can contribute to anxiety and fear.

Many people equate chemical reactions with irritated eyes, nose, or skin. If fumes are ingested, there may be gastrointestinal complaints. Indeed, this is often the case. More frequently, however, the symptoms are less obvious and include fatigue, laziness, forgetfulness, lack of concentration, headaches, assorted aches and pains, and swelling. Each person may react with different symptoms. Some will go on to develop palpitations, excessive perspiration, pallor, weakness, hyperactivity, panic, and phobias. Note that mental symptoms can and do occur without physical symptoms being present.

As one patient of mine recalls, "For no reason at all I would suddenly have a panic attack. I would shake, get "rubber" legs, sweat, have palpitations and a sensation of impending doom. I didn't know what to expect next, but I felt as though I were dying."

This statement came from a hairdresser whose hands were constantly exposed to dyes and other chemicals. Her main complaints were panic attacks, nightmares, unusual fears, and premenstrual syndrome. After a workup, it was determined that she was a chemically sensitive patient. She was told to wear gloves while using chemicals and to avoid chemicals altogether whenever possible. She was also placed on selenium, and B vitamins, including extra B and calcium. Her response was immediate: she ceased having nightmares; the panic attacks did not recur; and her premenstrual syndrome disappeared. Whenever she forgot her vitamins or had direct exposure to chemicals, however, her disorders temporarily returned; but as long as she took her supplements, she remained symptom-free. Of course, the patient could have changed her occupation, but such a step is usually impractical financially, and often adequate relief can be obtained by offsetting toxic effects.

One other postscript on this particular patient: Whenever she drank too much or indulged in excessive sweets, her symptoms would return in spite of the supplements. After this fact was pointed out, she learned to control her symptoms by simply reducing her intake of alcohol or sweets. The reason for the reaction is that sugar has a generally adverse effect on the immune system.

Dr. William Rea, M.D., a Texas clinical ecologist, introduced the concept of "total body stress load." Every individual has a limited capacity to handle stress, determined by his own genetic strength and life experiences. This stress load capacity is burdened by an accumulation of all the various stresses that the body experiences at any one time, be they environmental, emotional, or physical. Dr. Rea uses the analogy of a "rain barrel" filling with water. Once the "stress barrel" is full, it can overflow when even a small amount is added. In this manner, once our stress capacity is strained to the limit, even tiny quantities of inhaled or ingested chemicals can produce physical or mental symptoms.

Dr. Hans Selye is recognized as the father of modern stress theories. His view is that environmental stresses, whether infective, toxic, or emotional, can cause an alarm reaction in our bodies. If we can't avoid stress, then we have to adapt to it. When we are continuously forced to adapt to stress, we are compelled to use extra energy. This, of course, causes an additional drain on our energy and produces the chronic fatigue so familiar to those with allergies.

Dr. Stephen Levine, M.D., in his book *Antioxidant Biochemical Adaptation* (1984), uses the analogy of "interchangeable units" of stress. Since stress of any kind causes the body to react in pretty much the same way, it doesn't matter whether the units of stress are chemical or emotional—the reaction of the body will be identical.

Researchers have differing views of the biochemical-physical changes that result from stress. Some believe that the hypothalamus receives the brunt of the burden since this area of our brain is largely responsible for keeping our body in balance. Another theory is that a number of highly reactive free radicals are produced by oxygen in living systems. In this special state, oxygen is referred to as "partially reduced." Although oxygen is necessary for survival, this partially reduced form of oxygen can be extremely toxic to human tissue and thus can cause the symptoms attributed to stress.

In his book, Levine also mentions that stresses cause oxidative damage to bodily tissues. Normal oxidative conditions facilitate metabolic efficiency. Extremes in O_2 tension (hypoxic or hyperoxic) encourage electron leakage and oxygen-radical production, which is toxic to tissues. The possibility of tissue damage is balanced against the tissue's ability to exert antioxidative reactions.

Chemically sensitive patients are unable to tolerate inhaled or ingested chemicals at levels to which the general population is normally exposed. What may be an acceptable exposure level to one person can be damaging to another. Those who are oversensitive when exposed to even small amounts of offending chemicals will react by developing mental or physical disorders.

Some experts now think that up to 25 percent of the population is chemically hypersensitive, and many of these unsuspecting patients are labeled as hypochondriacs when they complain of numerous, unrelated symptoms. Chemically sensitive individuals, however, improve quickly as soon as they get relief from the offending substances. For example, I discovered that a patient of mine with a variety of physical complaints also experienced high levels of anxiety and occasional panic attacks.

This patient told me: "After I became aware of this thing called chemical sensitivity, I became aware of possible exposures that might set off my unexplained attacks of anxiety and fear. First, I discovered that my stove was slowly leaking enough gas to produce anxiety when I was in my home. I always wondered why I usually felt better when I was outside. I also noticed that newsprint, especially on my fingers, would make my nose itch and create a feeling of anxiousness. To my surprise, I also discovered that certain garments were related to panic attacks. Finally, I realized that it had more to do with the dye than the fabric, because I could wear the same fabric in other colors without incident."

Once an individual becomes aware of his sensitivities, he can be on the lookout for sources of trouble. Having catalogued his triggers, he can then control his symptoms either by avoidance or by the use of supplements that can block his reactions. However, when an individual becomes highly susceptible to chemicals, he will rarely, if ever, achieve a spontaneous cure. Becoming sensitive to one chemical also increases the chance of developing sensitivity to others, even in minute amounts. Dr. Rea has called this the "spreading phenomenon." There is no good explanation as to why it occurs, but it is well recognized among clinical ecologists that without intervention hypersensitivities become progressively worse.

Chemicals can act as a source of stress, altering the immune system so that even the smallest exposures will overtax the body. On the other hand, they may not have contributed to the initial weakening of the defense system, but may simply act as an additional burden which can tip the scale toward illness. Either way, chemicals can affect us negatively, and we must become aware of their relationship to mental disorders.

In Chapter 4 you will find methods of neutralizing these triggers and follow-up references for those who need professional help. The first step, as with so many problems, is to become aware of the possibilities, and to search for any and all connections that reasonably apply.

Trigger No. 12—Foods

Virtually any food can trigger a panic or anxiety attack. If the patient has no knowledge of these dietary effects, he will continue to eat foods that may be producing several negative reactions. Quite frequently, the foods we love the most are the ones doing us in and are the very ones we need to avoid. There has recently been much media attention focused on food allergies. It may have created some confusion, but for our purposes here, I want to assure you that anxiety and panic attacks can very definitely be caused by foods.

Around the turn of the century, doctors first began seriously to consider the idea that illness might be related to lowered resistance to internal disorders. At that time, immunology was only in its infancy. Even then, however, there were occasional reports of psychological disorders resulting from common foods.

What Is a Food Allergy?

The word *allergy* is derived from two Greek words meaning "altered reactivity." Allergists, however, are widely divided in their theories; some define allergy strictly as a reaction between antigens and antibodies, and others support the broader definition that allergies represent any overreaction of the body. Most of us relate them to pollens, dust, molds, and danders. These substances produce dramatic reactions which are easily charted in laboratory tests.

Pollens and dusts are further removed from us than foods. It's easier to accept an external cause, unrelated to our daily habits, than to acknowledge than an allergy might be triggered by a favorite treat. It's far more palatable to relate health problems to mold in the attic than to a beloved chocolate truffle!

Food allergies can cause all sorts of physical complaints, the most obvious being indigestion, gas, constipation, diarrhea, bloating, nausea, vomiting, colitis, and pain. We think of these symptoms as the body's efforts to reject some substance because of gastrointestinal irritation, and indeed, sometimes this is the case. But as we will see, it is far from being the most common form of reaction.

If pressed further about how the body reacts to foods, the average person might next consider skin changes. We've all heard that chocolate may cause acne or that milk can produce an allergic rash. But that's just the tip of the iceberg. There is practically no physical complaint that cannot be caused by hypersensitivity to foods. For example, I have seen a number of patients who have experienced complete relief from severe and intractable vaginal discharges after offending foods were identified and eliminated from the diet. Many of these patients had been to numerous doctors and tried a variety of drugs as well as other physical treatments.

Food allergies can also cause asthma, excessive urination, chronic bladder infections, unexplained bloating, irregular heartbeats, high blood pressure, arthritis, muscle spasms, chest and abdominal pains, fatigue, insomnia, weakness, headaches, irritability, anxiety, depression, and confusion. The list goes on and on. There is literally no possible symptom that cannot result from food sensitivities.

Food Allergies and Anxiety

Most, if not all, patients with high anxiety levels have overstressed immune systems, and an unknown number overreact to certain foods. Before treating patients for anxiety symptoms, I make an effort to determine if they have any food or chemical hypersensitivities. Once diagnosed, these triggers can be easily controlled, thus allowing the immune system, and ultimately the neurological system, to be relieved of excessive stress.

It is interesting to note that many of the drugs used to combat depression and anxiety also have antiallergic properties. Although orthodox medicine has not attributed any of their benefits to antihistamine effects, it may well be that these properties are contributing substantially to symptom relief.

Food As Triggers to Panic

Emotional symptoms top the list of allergic reactions to foods, and those reactions most definitely include panic attacks and phobias. As one patient explained, "Until I underwent food-allergy testing, I was not aware that tomatoes were linked to my anxiety attacks. If I ate anything with ketchup, or if I had a pizza, I would suffer an attack. Sandwiches and soups could also set me off. I never realized how many things contained tomatoes. I now avoid them at all costs."

And another patient laments, "Oranges seem to initiate my panic attacks, but I never realized it until I was tested. I've always loved oranges and used to eat them all the time. When I suffered from PMS, I would eat even more so I wouldn't give in to my cravings for sweets, and that only made things worse. Since I have learned about food allergies, I can now prevent some of these episodes."

Another young woman relates, "It seems like every time I eat any product containing wheat, I start to break down and cry, and I shake uncontrollably. I get pale and weak and think I'm going to die. It's hours before I can regain any sort of self-control."

WHAT CAUSES FOOD ALLERGIES?

Food is a more frequent cause of allergic reactions than most people realize. A large number of Americans, at one time or another, find themselves allergic to certain foods. Many of these cases start in childhood and continue as the patient matures. Three basic conditions contribute to the development of food allergies.

1. INHERITED TENDENCIES

Allergies may be inherited; frequently several family members are symptomatic. There have been reported cases of sensitivity to milk, fruit, vegetables, and fish that can be traced back two and three generations. One physician discovered egg sensitization in four generations of the same family. The stronger the history of family allergy, the earlier one might experience it. But although there often exists a family history of allergies, the absence of such a legacy does not necessarily mean that one is immune.

Some people believe that food allergies occur only among infants or small children. Adults don't expect to become allergic and commonly believe that, if they do, the condition will be temporary. Nothing could be further from the truth. The older one becomes, in fact, the more food allergies one is likely to develop, even in the later stages of life.

2. EXPOSURE

The more a person exposes himself to a specific kind of food, the more allergy-prone he will become. Certain ethnic groups consume large amounts of bread and milk products. Italians are famous for their pasta, cheese, and garlic bread, Hispanics for their cheese and tortillas, and all of those items contain yeast. As you might imagine, we find a high incidence of yeast and wheat allergies among these groups.

Too much exposure to one kind of food at one particular time may also overwhelm the immune system and trigger the allergic process. The combined assault of chemicals, excessive pollens, dusts, and molds with excessive intake of sugar, milk, yeast, or wheat can overload one's body to the breaking point.

Lack of variety in the diet is a widespread problem in American society. Fast-food chains have rapidly taken over our meal planning. The diet of the average American is becoming more and more repetitious. Hamburgers, fries, colas, tacos, candies, and sweets galore are all consumed by a society constantly on the move. These eating habits can lead to the pathological problems of allergy and addiction. But of all environmental exposures, we are probably more constantly exposed to repetitious foods than to any other substance. With such eating patterns so widespread, it is surprising that everyone doesn't develop addictive food allergies.

3. HEALTH AT THE TIME OF EXPOSURE

Quite frequently, patients claim that their allergies have begun after a serious illness or major psychological stress.

Some food allergy experts estimate that up to 90 percent of all Americans experience some form of food allergy. Even making a more conservative guess, the figure would certainly be over 50 percent. Addictions can grow stronger with time, and old addictions may stimulate new ones, creating a complex and ongoing problem.

Summary

There are many triggers to panic attacks. It's necessary to be able to identify and understand each particular trigger so that you can avoid or modify the attack before it starts. Even those who do not have full-blown panic, but only high-anxiety levels, should be aware of this phenomenon. Anxiety-prone people can be kept hyperactive and nervous by triggers in much the same way as those who have full-blown panic attacks. In Chapter 4, I will discuss methods of coping with these triggers, both with and without professional help.

4

General Treatment

Why do we have a special chapter on general treatment? Why not just list each treatment individually? The answer is that there are certain common factors that cross boundaries and are applicable to more than one anxiety. For example, food allergies are definitely triggers to panic and phobias of all varieties. It is much simpler to supply the treatment for this problem at the beginning of the book than to repeat it in every chapter. All of the general treatments in this chapter apply equally to each specific phobia. This chapter will also provide a foundation to help you develop a solid program for decreasing your anxiety levels. First, we'll deal with general concepts, then proceed to specifics.

IS SELF-HELP POSSIBLE?

Is it reasonable to expect to help oneself overcome illness? Since a number of research papers have indicated that self-help is quite efficacious for many patients, you may ask, "Is a therapist really necessary?" Naturally, professional counseling is beneficial in many cases, but for some patients, it may not be essential or even practical. For example, a 1973 study by Evans and Kellam, documenting an attempt to automate desensitization treatment, concluded: "The results show that clinically phobic patients can benefit just as well from automated therapy as from live therapy." Automated therapy is a preset program that patients can use by themselves.

Another paper that appeared the same year, "Self-Directed Desensitization for Agoraphobia," by Baker, Cohen, and Saunders, found that "Self-directed desensitization was found to be every bit as effective as standard desensitization which involves considerably more therapist time." Follow-up studies noted that patients in the study continued to improve after the research was completed. Interestingly, interviews with these patients developed the finding that most patients preferred to treat themselves rather than rely on someone else. Most felt they would not be as relaxed with another person.

Exposing oneself to the object of one's fear is the major element in this type of treatment, and it can be accomplished without a therapist. It is not important how the patient approaches the task, as long as it gets done. Frequent exposures eventually lead to desensitization, and desensitization means gradual loss of symptoms.

Who Should Rely on Self-Help?

Self-help, though valuable, is limited, and there are some for whom it is simply not appropriate. This list of questions will help you determine whether or not this type of therapy is right for you.

1. Are you seriously thinking of suicide or even homicide? If so, your illness is acute and immediate professional help is essential. Self-help can be practiced later on when your condition is stabilized.

2. Are you under the influence of alcohol or drugs a great deal of the time? If so, it's not advisable to attempt self-therapy. You need professional assistance and a strong support group to help combat this difficult problem.

3. Do you suffer from a serious physical illness such as asthma, heart disease, or poorly controlled diabetes? If so, do not attempt any form of self-help without your doctor's approval.

The Starting Point

First determine your present level of functioning.

1. How long have you had fears and anxieties? _____

_____

2. Have you undergone any form of therapy or counseling? _____

_____

3. If you discontinued therapy, how long ago? _____

_____

4. List all medicines that you take, including prescription, over-the-counter, and street drugs. _____

_____

5. Do friends and family members really understand your fears and worries? _____

_____

6. Do you feel you are coping adequately? _____

_____

7. What seems to help the most? _____

_____

8. What seems to make things worse? _____

_____

9. Do you now attend any support or therapy groups? _____

_____

10. Have you ever studied meditation or relaxation techniques?

_____

11. Have you ever kept a record of your fear patterns? _____

_____

12. What other books have you read on this subject? _____

_____

This is not a test. The point is for you to take the time to review, in an organized way, what has happened to you up till today. Now you have a record to refer to later should the need arise. You've also had a chance to put into words thoughts that may have only been vague shadows before. Clarification is always good. Let's move on.

Goals

Before you begin therapy for agoraphobia, for example, make a list of *clearly defined goals*. Don't say, "I want to go out more." Instead declare, "I want to go to the 7-11 store, four blocks from my house." Don't merely indicate a desire to be more sociable; decide that you will visit your old friend, Susie. If your aims are not precise, you can never be certain that you've attained a certain goal. Having a definite feeling of achievement builds your self-confidence, which further lowers your fears and encourages you to proceed onward. Take the time to be as clear and detailed in your answers as possible.

1. What is the first and most important problem that needs solving?

_____

My treatment goal is: _____

2. My next most important problem to solve is: _____

_____

My treatment goal is: _____

  3. My next most important problem to solve is: _____

_____

My treatment goal is: _____

  4. My next most important problem is: _____

_____

My treatment goal is: _____

_____

Keep a diary of your practice and achievements. Without a written log, it's sometimes difficult to keep track of your gradual improvement.

Setbacks and Failures

In the pages to follow there will be suggested exercises which can be used to help one begin to face these fears. Sessions can take from a few minutes to hours, and five or more sessions may be required to bring about changes.

It's easy to become depressed if you fail in some of your early ventures. Be assured that it happens to everyone; the process of change never occurs without setbacks. People learning to play a musical instrument go through periods when they don't seem to improve, no matter how hard they try. People attempting to lose weight have weeks when they can't shed a pound. These are called plateaus. The important thing is to go right on—for all plateaus can be broken through. Setbacks can last for hours or even weeks. If you thought you had conquered a certain situation, but old fears suddenly return, take heart. You've already proven that you can do it. The first time is always the hardest. You know you can do it again.

Simply use the same techniques, and you'll find that success comes more easily and more quickly the second time around. Through your practice, you will see you have the power to overcome problems more efficiently each time they occur. For a variety of reasons, all of us have "good" days and "bad" days. Not just in regard to phobias, but in all areas. Don't worry about it. One bad day is no indication of things to come—your goods days will be just around the corner.

Setbacks occur more often when you get overconfident and cut back on practice sessions. But should that happen, don't be discouraged. The best attitude is to erase completely any mistake or setback from your mind. That was yesterday's history. Today is all that's important. *You can just as easily predict the future by today's attitude as from a past failure.* It's present attitude that gives one the power to succeed.

You should also be aware that a disorganized and disturbed nervous system can be cantankerous, and may cause you to drift in and out of control. Even when you reach a stage of excellent control, there may be setbacks, for sudden attacks can resume at any time. Asthmatics are in a similar situation, for even when their breathing is essentially restored, they have good and bad days and may experience attacks under particular circumstances. Their breathing system is vulnerable and will never be perfect. With phobics, it's the nervous system that's sensitive, and it's never going to be totally normal. With this as a given, can you ever really expect to achieve peace of mind? The answer is an overwhelming yes. Why? Because an extremely high percentage of people with your condition have done it. Your chances of success are great if you just persevere and don't become discouraged.

Eliminate Important Triggers

Let's consider this example.

I was treating a patient for premenstrual syndrome (a hormonal imbalance), but we were getting only fair results using hormone therapy. The patient agreed to take some food allergy tests. It turned out that she was allergic to wheat, yeast, and milk, and her allergic reactions were exactly the same as the symptoms she had been experiencing as premenstrual problems: depression, anxiety, anger, mental confusion, and memory loss. When we discontinued the foods she was allergic to, her premenstrual symptoms completely disappeared. In other words, her symptoms were not caused by hormone imbalance. Very often, the symptoms experienced by panic and phobic patients are complicated by food allergies which exacerbate the problem. Unless the food allergies are identified and dealt with, nutritional supplementation may be only marginally effective. What applies to food allergies also holds true for chemical sensitivities. Here is a plan to control both food and chemical allergies if they are found to play an important role in fears and panic.

FOOD ALLERGY TEST AND TREATMENT

We have already discussed the triggering effect some foods have on individuals susceptible to anxiety symptoms. These reactions can be critical in serious cases and significant in mild to moderate cases. It's impossible, however, to know what foods you are allergic to without undergoing specific tests.

Who Should Be Tested for Food Allergies?

- If you suffer from agoraphobia, or if you experience extremely high levels of anxiety, you *should* consider testing.
- If you are a chronic worrier, obsessive-compulsive, overly shy, or an overresponder to stress, there is a likelihood that you are allergic, and you *may* wish to take the test.
- If you have only a simple phobia, such as an excessive fear of dogs, the test is useful but optional.

Testing

There are two tests that are necessary. You begin by eating one group of foods for four consecutive days, then consume the foods in the second group from the fifth day on, until you have tried all of the foods on the list.

RULES FOR TEST 1

1. Eat only one food, every three hours. The portion should be four times what is customary for an average meal. Drink only spring water and no other beverages. Salt is permissible, but no other foods or condiments. Test each item by eating enough within twenty minutes to make you feel full. Remember to wait at least three hours before eating the next food on the list.

2. You do not have to sample every food on this list. You may eat as many foods as you like but only one of the foods listed per meal. If you do not experience any reaction (see symptom list on pp. 70–71), then you may eat that food freely. This is called a negative reaction, and these foods may then be eaten along with any of the test foods that follow. By discovering these nonreactive foods, and adding them to your test foods, you can add both variety and content to your diet. If you do have a positive reaction to any particular food, you must *not* eat it again for the remainder of the testing period.

3. The foods on the list below are to be tested for four days only. Eat only the items on this list, carefully following the rules listed above. It is not necessary to test every food on this first list.

LIST 1

Vegetables	*Fruit*	*Protein*	*Nuts*
Broccoli	Watermelon	Lamb	Walnuts
Zucchini	Pears	Sole	Sunflower seeds
Squash	Cantaloupe	Haddock	
Cucumbers	Papaya	Salmon	
Celery	Blackberries	Halibut	
Brussels sprouts	Blueberries		

4. Take care in preparing all the test items. Ocean catches such as shrimp or fish should be broiled, baked, roasted, or steamed. Eat only raw vegetables and fruits. Don't add pepper, ketchup, mustard, sugar, honey, spices, vinegar, or other condiments. Nuts must be unprocessed.

5. Observe your reactions and write down each symptom, noting the exact time you tested the food and how soon the reactions occurred. You may experience some symptoms in the first twenty minutes. If you are reading, you may notice blurred vision. Most reactions appear within the first hour and usually will occur within four hours after eating. When each test is completed, review your records. If your reactions were severe, you will probably need to test further for chemicals, molds, and other substances, so make arrangements with a physician. If you don't wish to test yourself, but desire help, see Chapter 18 for the names of recommended professionals.

6. Keep a diary. If you don't have a written record, you might forget exactly which foods caused which of these symptoms.

    a. *Overactivity*—Nervousness, irritability, or arousal
    b. *Underactivity*—A sense of being sedated, boredom, tiredness, or sleepiness
    c. *Hunger*—An increased appetite
    d. *Personality changes*—A noticeable change in behavior, such as increased anger or fear

All of these reactions demonstrate a definite neurological allergy.

The symptoms can be described in two categories: "Subjective symptoms," or nonvisible sensations; and "Objective symptoms," or visible sensations. To provide examples, here is the symptom list used in my clinic.

Subjective Symptoms	Objective Symptoms
Nausea	Hiccups
Headache	Wheezing
Flatulence	Coughing
Itching	Sweating
Numbness	Herpes
Unsteady on feet	Burping
Dizziness	Flatulence
Fatigue	Change in skin color
Pain in parts of body	Rashes
Dry mouth	Hives
Thirst	Crying
Disturbance of smell	Rubbing eyes
Mental confusion	Runny nose
Visual disturbance	Circles under eyes

Subjective Symptoms	*Objective Symptoms*
Metallic taste	Lines under eyes
Itching of eyes	Blurred vision
Itching of mouth or throat	Spots before eyes
Ringing ears	Vagueness
Bloating	Faraway look
Joint pains	Rapid heartbeat
Pressure on chest	Bloating
Difficult breathing	Irritability
Swelling of mouth or throat	Flushing
Nose open or closed	Redness
Irritability	Eczema
Chilliness	Tenderness
Intoxication	Swelling
Increased appetite	Stuffiness
Mental alertness	Sinusitis

The most important symptoms we are searching for are a sense of panic, increased fears, increased anxiety, or any sensations which accompany panic attacks or phobias. If any of these reactions occur, you will need to neutralize them immediately in order to regain self-control.

How to Stop Food Reactions

If you have a reaction of any kind, you can quickly neutralize it with one of the following methods. Once a symptom has been reversed, wait at least one hour before doing further tests.

1. Prepare a neutralizer by mixing two parts baking soda with one part potassium bicarbonate. Both are available at your local pharmacy. Or you may simply use one teaspoonful of baking soda in a glass of water. If you have a reaction to any of the foods, drink the mixture immediately, and don't test again for at least an hour.

2. Another neutralizer is Alka-Seltzer. Take one tablet in a glass of water upon experiencing symptoms.

3. You may also use vitamin C crystals, two teaspoonfuls in a glass of water.

RULES FOR TEST 2

After completing Test 1 as directed, you are ready to deal with Test 2, which is the actual allergy elimination part of the diet. (The first four days were intended to purge your system of the allergens already present.) As you consume the foods on List 2, follow all instructions precisely.

1. Eat one food at a time, following the instructions for Test 1. Eggs should be hard boiled. Corn may be water packed or fresh on the cob. Boil cereals; you can test both wheat or oatmeal in cereal form. Boil barley in spring water to test for malt. When testing for sugar, place two tablespoonfuls in a glass of spring water. For yeast, use two cubes of Red Star baker's yeast in cold spring water. Note any possible reactions, physical or psychological.

2. If a reaction occurs, take any one of the three neutralizers recommended on pp. 71–72 with the List 1 foods. Wait one hour and test another food. You must try *all* the foods on List 2 once or more, noting all reactions.

3. If any item on List 2 produces symptoms, discontinue that food for the remainder of the diet.

It's important to describe all your reactions during the eating periods or shortly thereafter. Even subtle changes in your mental or physical state can be related to allergies.

Also note that during the initial four-day period when you abstain from your regular diet, you may experience feelings of withdrawal. This is normal and can be an indication of multiple food allergies. You will probably feel better after completing Test 1 because your system will be cleansed of allergens. To enhance the cleansing process, you may wish to add laxatives. If you are already sure that you are allergic to an item on List 2, you don't have to experiment with it; just make a note of your past experiences.

LIST 2 (to begin on the fifth day)

Milk	Corn	Tuna
Cheese	Baker's yeast	Oranges
Eggs	Soy beans	Peanuts
Beef	Tomatoes	Peanut butter
Chocolate	Potatoes	Shellfish
Wheat	Chicken	

After the Test

We have been testing for foods that might possibly trigger fears and anxieties. If you did not experience any symptoms, then food allergies are not your problem. On the other hand, if you *did* react, what do you do about the foods that acted as triggers?

How Do You Control Your Food Allergies?

1. Obviously, the obvious way to combat food allergies is to scrupulously avoid the offending items. But for how long? In the case of foods that cause very mild symptoms, twelve weeks of avoidance is usually long enough.

2. In the case of stronger reactions, allergy-producing foods ought to be avoided for six to nine months. After that time, they can be reintroduced to your diet on a twice-a-week basis. Certain foods are "fixed," that is, they are programmed into your system in such a way that they can never be freely eaten without symptoms.

3. If you crave these foods, you should read my book, *No More Cravings* (Warner Books, 1986), and apply its suggested techniques whenever your cravings are active.

4. Food allergies can be treated by physicians and clinical ecologists. Some allergists are also experienced in desensitization treatment.

5. In general, you should try to broaden your basic diet, instead of eating the same foods every day. Try rotating four or five variations at each meal. The more foods you rotate, the less likely you are to develop new allergies or rekindle old ones.

6. Nutritional supplements
   a. Take a good multivitamin. I recommend Nutra-Homo because it is complete in vitamins, minerals, and amino acids.
   b. Ascorbic acid, vitamin C powder. When vitamin C is taken on a regular basis, food allergy reactions become minimal. You'll have to discover what dose is best for you. I recommend to my patients one teaspoonful (4,000 mg) three times a day to start, and you may go up or down from there. Be sure to take extra potassium (100 mg), calcium (about 400 mg), and magnesium (about 200 mg), because vitamin C strips them from the body by a process called chelation.
   c. Digestive enzymes. There are several types; experiment and see which works the best for you. One group is derived from papaya, and another group is a combination of pancreatic enzymes and bile salts. Digestive enzymes taken with food help to break it down for easier digestion. When this happens, there is usually a dramatic decrease in allergy symptoms. Two tablets at each meal are standard.
   d. Desiccated liver tables. Dr. Marshall Mandel, in his book *5-Day Allergy Relief Symptoms* (Pocket Books, 1980), suggests the use of desiccated liver tablets. They can be obtained from any health food store and are relatively inexpensive. They can also be purchased from Rowl Chemical Company, West Palm Beach, Florida. Liver tablets are an excellent source of energy because they are high in B vitamins. If you take them in large amounts, you can reduce your multivitamin intake. I suggest six to twenty liver tablets per day for most patients, depending on individual needs.
   e. Vitamin B_6 is always necessary to help the body cope with allergies. I recommend 50 mg three times daily. Do not exceed 200 mg a day, for too much can produce toxic symptoms. Also, there are some individuals who may feel worse when taking B_6. If this happens, switch to paradoxyl-5-phosphate, a superior but more expensive form of the vitamin.

CHEMICAL SENSITIVITY TEST

This test will provide a general assessment of your chemical sensitivities. The more questions you answer yes to, the more likely you are to be chemically sensitive and therefore vulnerable to addiction.

	YES	NO
1. Do you strongly suspect you are chemically sensitive?	_____	_____
2. Are you bothered by natural gas from household stoves and washers?	_____	_____
3. Are you easily able to detect leaking gas?	_____	_____
4. Do certain fabrics bother you (cotton, silk, wool, linen, kapok, dacron)?	_____	_____
5. Are you bothered by certain kinds of rugs? What about curtains?	_____	_____
6. Do household cleaners affect you (soaps, detergents, scouring pads, bleach, Lysol, Pine-Sol, airwicks, cornstarch, furniture polish)?	_____	_____
7. Do you experience symptoms when the wind is blowing toward you from an industrial area?	_____	_____
8. Are you negatively affected by tap water?	_____	_____
9. Are you bothered by insect spray, moth balls or crystals, exterminator sprays?	_____	_____
10. Are you sensitive to gasoline or garage fumes?	_____	_____
11. Do you react to diesel smoke or auto exhaust?	_____	_____
12. Do you feel ill when exposed to lighter fluid?	_____	_____

                                        YES   NO

13. Do you suffer from the fumes of nail polish remover?

14. Are you sensitive to fresh newspapers?

15. Are you bothered by kerosene, metal, shoe polishes, or turpentines?

16. Do hand lotions, face creams, petroleum jelly, or mineral oil cause you to react?

17. Are you affected by burning wax candles, or auto or glass wax?

18. Are you sensitive to fresh tar or asphalt?

19. Do you react to carbon paper, typewriter ribbons, or ointments?

20. Are you bothered by dyes in clothing or shoes?

21. Do you react to cosmetics, such as lipstick, mascara, rouge, or powder?

22. Are you sensitive to any types of rubber?

23. Are you bothered by plastics or adhesives?

24. Does rubbing alcohol, varnish, lacquer, or shellac cause you to have symptoms?

25. Are you unable to drink alcohol?

26. Are you bothered by shampoos, perfumes, colognes, hair spray, or scented soaps?

27. Are you affected by air conditioners?

28. Do you react adversely to Christmas trees, evergreen decorations, pine, cedar, or other woods?

29. Are you sensitive to any medications?

Take an overview of the test and see how many yes answers you record. If you've replied yes on two or more of the questions, it's possible that you are chemically sensitive. If you said yes on five or more of the questions, you are very likely to fall into this category.

Personal Observations

If you are still uncertain, the next step is to observe closely *how* you react to the items you have marked. It might be helpful to keep a record of each response. After several weeks, a pattern should emerge which will help you determine whether or not you are chemically sensitive, to what degree, and to what substances. Any mental changes in the presence of these chemicals, such as confusion, forgetfulness, irritability, fatigue, depression, or the main symptoms dealt with in this book—feelings of panic or anxiety, agitation, hyperactivity, or hypoglycemic symptoms—are all positive signs of a chemical allergy.

Controlling Chemical Sensitivities

After completing the above test and charting your responses, you should now know whether or not you are abnormally sensitive. If the test suggests you are, the procedures listed below should provide some relief until you contact your physician for in-depth treatment. Unless you suffer only a mild sensitivity, self-help alone is inadvisable. If you suspect you have a problem but are not absolutely certain, you may confirm your suspicions by seeing a physician or by simply starting on the program listed below. If it turns out that you're not chemically sensitive, the treatment will be harmless and will, in fact, be beneficial to your immune system.

Short-Term Relief

1. Avoidance is always the first choice. Try to avoid contact with any item that causes a reaction. This is, of course, sometimes easier said than done. If avoidance is possible only some of the time, or logistically impossible, then go on to the next group of treatments.

2. If you have sudden unexpected contact with your allergen, take an Alka-Seltzer cold tablet, and do some deep, slow, relaxed breathing. Really oxygenate your lungs. Very often this will provide some immediate relief.

3. Certain nutritional supplements are also known to help patients develop resistance to chemical sensitivities.

   a. Selenium—400 micrograms daily. Begin with a much smaller quantity and gradually work up to this dosage. But be warned—you may be one of those individuals who are highly sensitive to selenium. Although you may require this mineral, you may not be able to tolerate even the smallest amount. Although selenium is important to the chemically sensitive patient, it *must* be used properly. The protocol for taking selenium can be obtained from Dr. Steven Levine, Ph.D., Nutra-Cology, Inc., P.O. Box 489, 400 Preda St., San Leandro, CA 94577-0489, telephone (415) 639-4572.

   If you react adversely to the selenium, don't try it again until you have contacted Dr. Levine or sought advice from a qualified nutritionist, and never exceed 400 micrograms daily.
   NOTE

   There are generally three reactions that chemically sensitive patients have to selenium.

   Group I—Slow, subtle improvement over a two-month period, with no immediate benefit. People in this group must be patient.

   Group II—Immediate improvement.

   Group III—These individuals experience an adverse reaction (general malaise, fatigue and weariness, irritability, mental confusion) to selenium or other nutritional items. In this case, it's necessary to dilute the selenium and start with a very small amount. Take your selenium bottle and put several drops in a glass of water. Add a teaspoon of this mixture into a second glass of water, and gradually work up to a larger dosage.

   b. Ascorbic acid powder or crystals—vitamin C is a powerful antioxidant and detoxifier, and it can be useful to the chemically allergic individual. The proper dose will vary from person to person, so you'll have to experiment in order to find the correct amount. Some clinical ecologists suggest starting with a teaspoon, which contains about 4,000 mg of vitamin C. If there are no side effects, increase to two or more teaspoons daily. Remember, whenever you take large doses of vitamin C, be sure to add extra potassium (100 mg), calcium (400 mg), and magnesium (200 mg) to your diet, because vitamin C interferes with their absorption. Vitamin C powder may also be obtained from Nutra-Cology (address on p. 78), or from your local health food store.

c. Zinc citrate or picolinate—25 mg daily. Occasionally it is necessary to increase the dose to 200 mg, but be sure you never exceed that amount, because too much can suppress the immune system and have an adverse effect on copper and selenium. Even if your multivitamin contains 25 mg of zinc, it's still wise to take an extra tablet daily, because some multivitamins offer zinc in a form that is not easily absorbed.

d. Take a good multivitamin. I prefer a brand called Nutra-Homo because it contains a broad spectrum of vitamins, minerals, and amino acids in a form that is absorbed slowly. Nutra-Homo Inc. is based in Los Alamitos, California, but your local health food store can order it for you. You should be aware, however, that too large a dose of these vitamins can make you feel nervous or hyper. It's best to begin with half a teaspoonful of the powder and work up. If you use tablets, the dose recommended by the manufacturer is about ten daily. A good multivitamin will keep your basic nutrition in balance while you start to recover. If you are sensitive to chemicals and already have found a good multivitamin that you tolerate well, by all means stay with it.

e. Vitamin B_6 is essential for most chemically sensitive individuals. The best form of this is paradoxyl-5-phosphate, but it is quite expensive. Sometimes, however, the cost is well worth it because many individuals cannot utilize the form of B_6 that exists in most commercial products. If you are taking B_6 but have not observed any benefits, I suggest you give paradoxyl-5-phosphate a try. One 50 mg tablet three or four times a day is the usual dose. But a word of caution: More than 200 mg on a daily basis can be toxic to the nervous system, although in the instance of sudden, overwhelming exposure to offending chemicals, you might benefit from taking an immediate extra 100 mg.

f. Amino acid supplements have been covered on pages 38–45.

g. Pantothenic acid—4 500 mg capsules or tablets will help combat all forms of stress. It supports the adrenal gland as well as potentiating all of the B vitamins, including B_1. A good deal of pantothenic acid is required to protect the body, so the amounts given in the average multivitamin are generally inadequate.

h. Special formulations of antioxidants, which include dimethylglycine, are available from Nutra-Cology or your local health food store. These supplements are of great help to chemically sensitive persons. The number of tablets needed daily depends on the manufacturer's formula and personal requirements.

Long-Term Relief

1. Injection therapy—some chemically susceptible individuals who are sensitive to common house dust may achieve symptom relief with an injection of dust extract, because there is an interrelationship between dust, molds, and chemicals. Some physicians desensitize their patients with the actual allergy-producing chemical.

2. Treat all food or pollen allergies, because they ultimately suppress the immune system and restrict chemical tolerance levels.

3. If you have a furnace, air conditioner, gas appliance, rug, or any other household item that is making you feel ill, it should be repaired or replaced, so that chemical stress is minimized.

4. Any areas of your house with excess mold or dust should be well cleaned because these two substances potentiate chemical sensitivities.

5. Chemicals often contaminate foods, so you may need to peel fruits and vegetables, consume only health store products, and switch to foods less likely to have chemical exposure, such as fish or frozen seafoods. If you eat meat, remove as much of the fat as possible, eat unprocessed nuts, and use only cold-pressed oils.

Summary of Short-Term Relief

Most important:

1. Selenium, 400 mcg
2. Ascorbic acid powder, 4,000 mg and up
3. Zinc, 25 to 200 mg
4. One good multivitamin
5. Vitamin B_6, 200 mg
6. Pantothenic acid, 1,500 mg daily
7. Antioxidant formula
8. Essential fatty acids with vitamin E

You should be aware that chemically sensitive patients generally tend to get worse. If you are sensitive to one chemical, you are likely to slowly develop other allergies as well.

Up to this point, you have organized yourself to begin a program of self-help treatment. You know what your goals are, and you are fairly sure you have detected and eliminated the foods and chemical antigens you are sensitive to. These are two of the most important triggers to panic and phobias. Now here are some other methods that can help you.

COPING TECHNIQUE NO. 1—
PARADOXICAL INTENTION

I have included this method of coping here in the chapter on general treatment because it is useful in treating almost all forms of anxiety, regardless of the nature of the fear. I will refer to this technique often in the following chapters.

There are certain responses to stress that most people experience to some degree, but some of them are more severe in anxiety patients. Have you noticed any of the following?

- Trying to control anxiety only makes it more intense (fighting your symptoms is the worst thing you can do).
- Anticipating anxiety can precipitate an attack.

- Excessive attention to one's own performance interferes with what one wants to do. The harder you try to sleep, the more difficult it becomes. The harder you "try" at sex, the more problems you create.

It is necessary to change these self-defeating scenarios. The aim is to stop trying to eliminate the symptoms of anxiety and instead strive to *create* them. The magic behind this theory is that the more you consciously try to intensify your symptoms, the weaker they will become. By making an effort to experience the very symptoms you have been trying to avoid, you are enabled to bring them under control. Anxieties are intensified by your attempt to fight or to avoid them, so this technique works by taking the reverse approach.

Principles of the Treatment

1.   The symptom is not avoided but, rather, faced directly through intentional effort.

2.   A large part of the total anxiety experience is caused by efforts to exert control. These attempts merely heighten fear and panic.

3.   The idea is to cease fighting, submit to the feelings, and deliberately try to intensify them.

4.   You can practice in your home by first summoning up thoughts that trigger anxiety, then gradually increasing their frequency and intensity.

5.   Practice the problem behavior routinely rather than allowing it to occur sporadically. Command the problem behavior to display itself.

6.   During a panic attack, first focus your mind on that part of your body most affected by anxiety. Is it your muscles, your stomach, your brain, throat or lungs, trembling hands, or your heart? Choose the worst area and try to define your exact feelings. Are you jittery, fearful, anxious? Identify your chief reaction, then concentrate all your attention on accentuating it. If you consider, for example, your tremor to be an eight on a scale of one to ten, then try to double

its intensity. Usually, the tremor will worsen for about thirty seconds, then completely disappear. If it returns, repeat the exercise, but try even harder. If there is another area of your body that is also tense and anxious, repeat the same procedure. First try to understand it, and then attempt to mimic it as an actor does, making it many times larger than life. You may find that the symptom rarely recurs, but if it does, dramatize and exaggerate it. Eventually, you will wipe it out forever.

Don't withdraw from discomfort. Instead, attack it with everything you've got. Attack with anger—decisively. Make fear *your* victim. It's had you on the run all this time; now you can turn the tables. Become the one in power.

One therapist asked a patient who was concerned about having a coronary during a panic attack to try as hard as he could to speed up his heartbeat to the point of cardiac arrest. The doctor was not subjecting his patient to risk, for this individual has a perfectly normal heart and could not, under any circumstances, comply with the request. As the man soon discovered, his attempts to create a heart attack not only failed, they quickly reduced his rapid heartbeat and ended his anxiety. In order to achieve long-term results, he was told to try to create a heart attack several times a day, on a regular schedule.

Here is another variation of Paradoxical Intention you can use.

- Make up a list of ten fearful situations, ranging them in order from the least threatening to the most threatening.
- Take the first three, and expose yourself to those conditions while practicing your Paradoxical Intention procedure.
- Record the degree of anxiety felt before and after each session.
- Review your progress at the end of each week.
- Pay attention and accentuate any anxiety during the exposure. Don't allow yourself to withdraw from any situation when you experience discomfort.
- Continue on down the list.

COPING TECHNIQUE NO. 2—RELAXATION

Relaxation can benefit chronically anxious patients in a number of ways. It is an active coping skill and not a passive retreat. Any procedure that interrupts the chain of anxious responses is of help and may be very beneficial for specific situational anxieties. After learning relaxation techniques, you can use this method to combat stressful situations.

Although relaxation has been a mainstay for some forms of therapy, it is not necessarily for everyone. Before you go any further, answer these questions:

- Do you think you will be able to relax?
- Do you think you will follow the program?
- If not, do you think you could make the necessary adjustments that would enable you to follow the program?
- Do you think your efforts will make a difference?

If your answers are mostly positive, then you probably will be helped by this anxiety-coping method, so read on and begin the exercise that follows. If, on the other hand, your answers are mostly negative, then you may wish to pursue other coping strategies.

Whichever category you fall into, it's important to know that relaxation is not essential to success. Each patient learns how to relax at a different rate. For some, the process of learning to relax might take longer than the entire process of curing the phobia. Some people can learn how to relax in an hour, while others might require six to ten hours or more. If you wish, you can begin desensitization or some other treatment technique before you have completely learned to relax. You can do both simultaneously.

What level of relaxation are you trying to reach? Deep muscle relaxation, or a feeling of calmness or mental relaxation? It's much easier to achieve a feeling of calmness than to learn individual muscle relaxation control. The feeling of calmness will serve you just as well as muscle control, and can be achieved in much less time.

A Technique for Attaining Inner Mental Calm

Sit in an easy chair and close your eyes. For twenty minutes imagine a pleasant mental image, such as a warm, peaceful, summer day, or picture yourself as a leaf, quietly and gently floating down a stream. You must get so deeply into the scene that you feel you're actually there. Experience each of the sensations with your eyes, your ears, your skin temperature, and your sense of smell. At the end of twenty minutes, if you have succeeded, you should feel very relaxed.

You must practice this mental relaxation daily for at least thirty days in order to make it a viable tool. During the day, when you have a free moment, try to reproduce that quick calming image. When your technique becomes strong and controllable, it can prevent you from escalating into a full-blown panic attack.

Monitor Your Anxiety

To monitor your anxiety effectively, you must keep a diary. Self-monitoring is just as important as learning relaxation. You must become consciously aware of all anxieties present and determine how you are coping with each one.

Deep Muscle Relaxation

If you would prefer to use the classical form of relaxation, consider buying one of the tapes that are available from a number of companies. You could also record your own voice and play it back, or simply follow a mental script. Either would be good for a start. Pre-record the script below on a tape recorder, then go into a quiet room, sit in a recliner or comfortable chair, close your eyes, and begin the exercise.

RELAXATION OF ARMS (time: 4–5 minutes)

Settle back and get comfortable . . . let yourself relax . . . just let go. . . . Now, as you relax, clench your right fist, that's it—tighter and tighter, making sure that you maintain the tension. Now, feel the tension in your fists and forearms . . . relax. Let your fingers, hands, and arms become loose, and notice the difference in your feelings . . . now let yourself go and try and become more relaxed all over. Once more, clench your fists tightly. Hold it, and notice the tension again. Let go, again relax . . . straighten your fingers out, and be aware of the difference. Clench your fists again while the rest of your body relaxes . . . tighter and tighter, feel the change.

Now relax your hands and forearms again . . . bend your elbows and tense your upper arms, tense them harder and harder. Then, straighten out your arms, let them relax, and experience the relaxation totally. Let the relaxation come over you. Once more: Tense your upper arms. Hold the tension for ten or fifteen seconds, then relax to the best of all your ability.

Each time, observe your feelings when you tense up and when you relax. Now, tense the muscles along the back of your arms; feel that tension ... and now relax. Take a break, get comfortable. Let the relaxation take over. Your arms should feel heavy as you let go ... feel that tension ... and unwind. Even when your arms feel fully relaxed, try to achieve deeper and deeper levels of relaxation.

RELAXATION OF FACIAL AREA, NECK, SHOULDERS, AND UPPER BACK (time: 4–5 minutes)

Let the muscles throughout your body become loose and limp. Settle back quietly and comfortably. Wrinkle up your forehead ... tighter, tighter ... then relax and feel your forehead become smoother as the relaxation continues. Frown and wrinkle your forehead once more. Next, close your eyes tighter and tighter ... after five seconds, relax your eyes. Repeat the tightening of eye muscles, then relax, three or four times.

Now clench your jaws, clamping your teeth together ... now relax your jaws. Repeat this several times. Open your mouth slightly, press your tongue hard against the roof of your mouth ... now, relax your tongue. Repeat this several times. Next, purse your lips, tighter and tighter ... relax the lips. Relax all the muscles in your face, your forehead and scalp, eyes, jaws, lips, tongue, and throat.

Turn your attention to your neck muscles. Tense them as tightly as you can ... now relax them. Rest a moment, then tense up again. Repeat this four times. Now relax yourself all over. Shrug your shoulders, hold the tension, then drop your shoulders and feel the relaxation in your neck and shoulders. Shrug your shoulders again and repeat this several times. Allow the relaxation to penetrate deeply into your shoulders and carry on into your back muscles. Now relax your neck and throat, then your jaws and other facial areas. Relax deeper, deeper, deeper ... ever deeper.

RELAXATION OF CHEST, STOMACH, AND LOWER BACK (time: 4–5 minutes)

Relax your entire body to the best of your ability. Feel heavy, then relaxed. Breathe in deeply and slowly, then relax and exhale, slowly.

Take deep breaths. Feel relaxed all over. Inhale deeply and hold your breath, filling your lungs. Feel warm all over. Now exhale, let your chest totally relax, let all the tension out. Continue relaxing and breathe deeply and slowly. Repeat this four or five times. Now, let the relaxation move to your back, shoulders, neck, and arms. Let go . . . let go. Be heavy and relaxed. Now your stomach area; tighten your stomach muscles, make them as hard as you can. Now relax. Let the muscles relax. Once more, tighten your stomach muscles. Hold the tension, then relax. Repeat this four or five times.

Search your body for tensions . . . let go of all muscle tightness anywhere in your body. Now turn your attention to your lower back. Tighten the muscles in your back, making it as tense as possible. Move the tension along your spine. Now relax the lower back . . . keep the rest of your body as relaxed as possible. Relax even more, deeper and deeper. Relax your lower back, your upper back, your stomach, chest, shoulders, arms, and facial area. Deeper and deeper, heavier and heavier, more and more relaxed.

RELAXATION OF HIPS, THIGHS, AND CALVES
(time: 4–5 minutes)

Let go of all tensions and relax. Tighten your buttocks and thighs. Now relax your thighs and buttocks; pressing down, tighten them again as hard as you can . . . relax completely. Wait a second . . . straighten your knees and flex your thigh muscles again . . . keep them tense. Now relax your hips and thighs. Repeat this three or four times. Then tighten your calves and feet. Keep them tense. Now relax them. Tighten your toes . . . relax them. Now let yourself relax still more, all over. Relax your feet, ankles, calves and shins, knees, thighs, buttocks, and hips.

COMPLETE BODY RELAXATION

Feel the heaviness of your lower body as you relax still more. Now relax your stomach, waist, and lower back. Relax more and more. Feel that relaxation all over. Relax your upper back, chest, shoulders, and arms, right down to the tips of your fingers. Relax more and more, deeper and deeper, heavier and heavier. Relax your throat; relax your neck and your jaws and all your facial muscles. Relax your entire body and keep it that way for a while. Go deeper and deeper.

You can become twice as relaxed as you are, merely by taking in a really deep breath and slowly exhaling. Keep your eyes closed. Be aware only of sounds: listen for voices, for traffic noise, now the wind or air conditioner and minor sounds. Listen to your own breathing, and feel yourself become heavier. Take in a long, deep breath and let it out slowly. Feel how heavy and relaxed you have become.

Now, completely relaxed, you should feel unwilling to move a single muscle in your body. Think how much effort it would take to raise your right arm. As you think about raising it, can you notice tensions that might have crept into your shoulder and your arm? You may decide not to lift the arm at all and go right on relaxing. See how the tension has all but gone. Feel how totally relaxed you are. Stay in this state of relaxation as long as you wish. When you finally decide to get up, count backwards from four. You should then feel fit and rejuvenated, wide awake, and calm.

An Alternative Method

An alternative method of relaxation is autogenic training. Visualize one part of your body, hold the image, and relax the corresponding part of your body. For example, get a clear picture of your right hand, see the outline of the fingers, the color of the skin, the wrinkles on the knuckles. Now relax your right hand as you concentrate on it. Keep the image in your mind all the time. Then, try to see your right forearm in your mind's eye. Continue this with all parts of the body.

DRUGS AND ANXIETY

Although this book stresses nutrition, in severe cases drugs are necessary as a first step in bringing symptoms quickly under control. Later you can decrease or discontinue them as nutrition and behavioral therapy take effect. Even if drugs do not play a role in your treatment, it is wise for you to be familiar with them, because they are a part of traditional treatments for this disease.

Propranolol

The drug propranolol is a beta-adrenergic blocking agent. It has been used successfully to control fear since 1965, and both anecdotal and research papers have referred to its efficiency in treating a wide range of anxiety symptoms. It appears to be a remarkably safe medication.

Although it effectively calms brain anxiety, propranolol's most important function is to quiet the overstimulated involuntary nervous system by alleviating palpitations and rapid heartbeat without sedating the patient. It also eliminates low blood pressure associated with panic attacks as well as hyperventilation. (One of the strongest tendencies of panic patients is to overbreathe during episodes of stress.) These adverse reactions, both of the brain and the body, are suppressed by the propranolol, thus reducing associated symptoms. Chest discomfort, muscle tension, and depression also decrease.

Propranolol has little potential for abuse and produces fewer side effects than other frequently prescribed medications. The only disadvantage is that it does not seem to work for everyone. It is a potent medication and requires a prescription. Patients with asthma, heart disease, slow pulse, and reliance on certain drugs are not good candidates for treatment with the drug. Possible side effects for users include fatigue, depression, gastrointestinal disturbances, and rashes. Some patients simply report lacking a general sense of well-being.

Tranquilizers

Most of these drugs belong to the benzodiazepine family, which includes Xanax, Tranxene, Librium, Valium, Paxipam, Ativan, Serax, and Centrax, and are used to control anxiety, muscle spasms, seizures, and epilepsy. They are by far the most widely prescribed drugs in the world.

Since their introduction more than 20 years ago (Librium was the first), their usage has steadily increased. In Canada, it has been estimated that each year ten percent of the general population receives a prescription for one of these drugs, while hospital patients have a usage of thirty percent. These figures are representative of most Western countries.

According to a 1979 book, *Phenomenology and Treatment of Anxiety*, these drugs are prescribed by psychiatrists for mental disorders in about thirty percent of all cases. In 1975, the Food and Drug Administration placed them on the restricted lists, for even low doses can produce physiological and psychological dependence.

The main function of these drugs is to ostensibly mitigate anxiety during the acute phase of an illness. While some cases of anxiety may be transient, agoraphobics, for example, have symptoms which can last for years, making such treatment highly questionable. Some doctors have subscribed to the idea that benzodiazepines may be preferable to the endless suffering of chronic panic, but frankly, if there are other choices—why not explore them?

Benefits of Antianxiety Drugs

Present-day antianxiety drugs are reliably effective. They rapidly calm even the most severe cases of anxiety, often without excessive side effects, making them a useful tool for the physician. Both patients and doctors feel that these drugs restore control over a "monster," thus providing a quick, easy solution.

Another advantage of such drugs is that they do not interfere with other methods of treatment, such as psychotherapy, behavior therapy, or group therapy. When the drugs are used for a short time while other therapies are being instituted, theoretically, the patient has the best chance of recovery. A number of reports have suggested that maximum period of use for these drugs should be about four months, but most doctors prescribe them for nine months to one year.

Disadvantages of Antianxiety Drugs

While these medications can produce an assortment of side effects, they are rarely serious. Probably the most immediate danger comes from their interaction with other drugs, particularly alcohol and narcotics. Elderly patients with slower metabolisms are especially sensitive. These problems aside, the greatest danger is the possibility of addiction.

Benzodiazepines, while often initially considered a godsend, can backfire into a nightmare if used improperly. They can be extremely addicting, both psychologically and physically, with physiological dependence occurring after long-term use of even low doses. Withdrawal triggers anxiety, insomnia, irritability, and tremors, in addition to the return of the original anxiety at a higher level. Withdrawal from larger amounts is similar to stopping heroin "cold turkey." Symptoms include pain, sweating, and trembling, up to and including grand mal seizures. This "rebound anxiety" can occur if patients are withdrawn from the drug after as little as three or four weeks of usage.

Today's newest antianxiety "wonder" drugs are considered spectacular in their ability to control symptoms, but they can be extremely addictive and difficult to discontinue. "Rebound anxiety" after withdrawal can be severe. Even slow withdrawal is difficult and sometimes impossible because these drugs become a cherished crutch. I've found that the most effective approach for patients who are already on tranquilizers is to begin a nutritional program and allow the benefits of the supplements gradually to replace the tranquilizer.

If a patient is too distraught to wait for the results of proper nutrition, then he *must* temporarily be placed on these medications until such a time as he can function without them. One method of treating or preventing withdrawal is to take niacinamide, 500 to 1,000 mg, with 50 mg of B_6, three times a day, while reducing the dosage of the tranquilizer by a third each week.

Benzodiazepines are sometimes called "minor tranquilizers," but their side effects, when they occur, are not minor. One of the most serious is loss of memory, which may significantly interfere with the learning of new material. These drugs may disturb the way we think and organize our thoughts. We can see brain wave abnormalities develop in people using these drugs, so it goes without saying that they could be quite a problem in children.

It has also been reported that some patients develop an increasing number of hates and dislikes. As these hatreds develop, more and more people are chosen for the patient's "hit list," until finally the symptoms escalate into full paranoia. In some cases, individuals even become dangerously aggressive and violent.

These drugs should not be used in the treatment of normal anxiety, such as everyday stress. Many people swallow them casually, unaware of their potential for producing major side effects in addition to mental and physical dependency.

If I can get patients early enough, before they become too drug-habituated, they will only need to rely on medication for a short time. Drugs were not designed to be a permanent part of one's life. Problems occur when no other form of therapy is administered, because eventually the drugs have to be discontinued.

There is always a temptation to overuse something that makes you feel good. It's normal to have ups and downs, but some people prefer to float through life, oblivious to all pain. Abusers will tend to use these medications when confronted with even the slightest amount of frustration or discomfort. Although instructed by their physicians to use medication only for *acute* anxiety, they will begin to use it to avoid normal, day-to-day problems, thus creating a dangerously vicious cycle.

No one can deny the usefulness of these drugs for short-term treatment of anxiety symptoms. But it should be emphasized once again that they only relieve the symptoms produced by the psychological and environmental factors that trigger anxiety. They do not have any effect on basic personality problems. If other techniques are not used concurrently, then there is little hope that the drugs will be of any real benefit, for their long-term value is practically nil. The relapse rate after these drugs' discontinuance has been found to be 90 percent.

Antidepressants and Phobias

For more than twenty years, agoraphobic patients have been treated with antidepressants to ameliorate their panic attacks. Nonagoraphobic patients who suffer from high fear levels and numerous phobias have also been successfully treated with this family of drugs. However, simple phobias such as a fear of heights do not tend to respond to antidepressants.

There are two major groups of antidepressants: tricyclics and monoamine oxidase inhibitors. The tricyclics block the area where the messenger (neurotransmitter) touches the nerve to excite it. The monoamine oxidase inhibitors work in a different way, by knocking out the chemicals that, in excess, destroy the messengers that stimulate the nerves. These drugs are highly potent, may produce many adverse side effects, and can interact strongly with each other as well as with other drugs, creating such symptoms as blurred vision, dry mouth, impotency, urine retention, constipation, and low blood pressure. Long-term effects may include irregular heartbeat, jaundice, neuropathy, confusion, and permanent tremors. The monoamine oxidase inhibitors have the added disadvantage of raising the blood pressure to acute levels when certain foods are eaten. Cheese, red wines, sausage, chocolate, and beer are among the foods that must be scrupulously avoided, along with certain drugs.

While experience shows MAO inhibitors to be useful in the treatment of the more intense types of anxiety, patients should be aware that there may be considerable discomfort and substantial risk.

The drug imipramine, one of the antidepressants in this family, has been particularly effective in the treatment of fears and anxiety. A dosage of 100 to 300 mg daily has been successful in controlling alcoholism in high-anxiety patients, and it has also proved very useful in the inhibition of panic attacks (Zitron, Klein, and Woerner 1978), as well as being a good assist to behavioral therapy.

Clonidine, the Antihypertensive

This drug, in addition to lowering blood pressure, is also used as a sedative. It has a strong antianxiety effect and has proven beneficial in the treatment of anxiety, panic, and phobias. It has fewer side effects than benzodiazepine and is nonaddictive, making it an excellent drug in many instances.

Antihistamines

Dr. Harold N. Levinson, M.D., in his book *Phobia-Free* (M. Evans 1986) recommends the use of antihistamines to stabilize inner-ear problems which he believes are responsible for many cases of panic and phobia. I would like to support him in his efforts to use less toxic and less addictive medicines whenever possible. Antihistamines such as Benadryl, Phenergan, and Atarax are relatively nontoxic to most patients, with the primary side effects being nothing more serious than a dry mouth and drowsiness.

Antinauseants

Dr. Levinson also recommends Antivert, Marezine, Dramamine, Vistaril, and Transderm-scop, all of which depress nerve activity in the inner ear, and consequently help to control panic and phobias. Like antihistamines, these drugs generally produce no worse side effects than a dry mouth and mild drowsiness, and, if effective, are an excellent alternative to the more toxic medications previously mentioned.

Drugs in Combination with Other Therapies

The more intense the anxiety, the more necessary is the use of drugs, at least initially. While medications have a number of negative side effects, they are the only real method of taming symptoms that are out of control. If the physician who treats a patient is knowledgeable about pharmacology, he will use the least toxic drugs that will serve the purpose. Once symptoms are under control, he should direct the patient toward other methods of treatment and minimize the use of any drugs that have multiple side effects and a potential for abuse.

While still on medication, patients can begin nutritional and/or behavioral therapy, which may eliminate the necessity for drugs altogether. Once these other approaches to panic and phobias become effective, the patient, under his doctor's direction, can gradually decrease his medication until he seldom, if ever, needs to rely on it. Individuals with lower levels of anxiety may never require medication at all and may be able to get immediate relief with nutritional and behavioral therapy.

Summary

I hope that by this time you have become well enough organized to start on your self-improvement program. Your food or chemical allergies should now be under control (if you have followed the directions properly). Psychologically, you will be aided by either or both of the two excellent coping techniques described. Paradoxical Intention is the easiest to learn and is very effective. The relaxation technique may take longer to master than other methods, but its value has been well proven. Now you can turn to the particular chapter that most closely relates to your own individual problem.

PART
2

CONQUERING
THE MAJOR FEARS

5

How to Conquer Agoraphobia

Agoraphobia, *Ag-o-ra-foh-bi-a*, is a difficult word to pronounce and a nearly impossible disease to live with. Simply defined, it is a morbid fear of open spaces, but to understand the disorder fully, one must be aware of its complexities.

Agoraphobia is a devastating disease and one that can be as incapacitating as psychosis. Categorized as a neurosis—a partial personality disorder—agoraphobia is not just a garden-variety form of anxiety that most of us deal with at one time or another. Rather, it is a crippling malady that can affect every area of a person's life.

As one patient told me, "I remember walking up the aisle in the market, and suddenly everything around me seemed unfamiliar. It was like a dream. I felt panic welling up inside me, but somehow I managed to go on with my shopping. As my anxiety worsened, I began to feel strangely unreal, almost as if I were watching myself in some terrifying movie. A woman passed by with her shopping cart, and I felt an urge to ask her, 'Am I really here?'

"With great difficulty, I continued on, but by now I was beginning to sweat, my hands were trembling, and my heart was pounding against my chest. I felt like I was on the verge of total insanity. My instincts told me to get home, but I was afraid if I started to run, I would completely lose control, so I moved slowly, holding on to anything near me. I only know that once inside my house, I broke down and cried for hours.

"The experience was so terrifying I didn't go out again for several days. When I finally did manage to visit my sister, I insisted that my mother come with me. Once there, I couldn't cope with her children and soon had a mild panic attack. This time I thought it was my heart, and I was sure I was going to die. As I fought to maintain consciousness, my sister wanted to call the paramedics, but my mother remained calm and reassuring, and somehow managed to get me home. After that experience, I refused to go out alone, and even when accompanied by someone else, my excursions were terribly difficult. Not only did I suffer from these panicky semi-fainting spells themselves, but I soon began to live in constant dread of their recurrence."

THE SYMPTOMS ARE SEVERE

This is a very simple and common example of how a person might first experience the symptoms of agoraphobia. The initial sensations are so severe, profound, and overwhelming that sufferers often fear for their life. Symptoms such as a fast-pounding heart, palpitations, shortness of breath, sweating, and dizziness are indeed similar to those of a heart attack, thus giving credibility to the feeling that something terrible is about to happen.

Most people initially conclude that they are either dying of a heart attack or losing their sanity. Unless one knows something about panic disorders, these are not illogical conclusions. And to make matters worse, the overpowering anxiety and fear that accompany such episodes often precipitate the beginning of a vicious cycle, as the fear of these attacks actually begins to trigger them.

The First Attack

The first attack may occur anywhere, in a shopping mall or on a street, in an elevator, or even at home. Future attacks are completely unpredictable and can happen anywhere at any time, causing the patient to feel constantly apprehensive. The fear of embarrassment, of fainting or nearly fainting in public, becomes overwhelming. Eventually, the patient becomes afraid to go anywhere or do anything.

Agoraphobics all react differently to their attacks; many want to hold on to someone for support, while others make the mistake of trying to fight the symptoms, which only increases their intensity and duration. Simply "giving in" to the episode seems to be the best approach, much like riding out a storm or a riptide.

Agoraphobia can be intermittent. A patient may go for months or even years without a panic attack, only to have them suddenly return. The agoraphobic is a prisoner in a body that can, at any time, become completely disorganized.

COMMON FEATURES OF AGORAPHOBIA

Some of the more common features of the disease follow:

The Fear of Leaving One's Home Fear of Going into Streets, Shops, or into Crowds

"The thought of leaving the house would throw me into a state of total frenzy," recalls one patient. "I was completely paralyzed. A sense of impending disaster made it impossible for me to speak; my heart would pound, and I could hardly breathe."

And from another patient, "Just after I left the house, it hit me. I wanted to run. A pervasive feeling of anxiety swept over me. My mouth was dry and I began to sweat. I had palpitations. My neck became tense, and I felt like throwing up."

Anticipatory Anxiety

Often called the "fear of fear," this phenomenon results from constant worry about having a panic attack.

"I couldn't stop thinking about how horrible the last attack was," says one young woman. "I was embarrassed and humiliated. The more I thought about it, the more anxious I became. The very thought that I might have an attack in public would nearly cause me to go over the edge."

Still another patient confides, "Panic suddenly struck and I had an overwhelming feeling of faintness—a terrible sensation of impending doom. I knew I must get home, but my legs were weak and useless—they seemed unable to carry me. My pounding heart wanted to crash through my chest."

Depersonalization

The feeling that one's existence is not real. "The world looked dark, distant, and surrealistic. I was detached from it. Everything was so far away, and I seemed to be going in and out of reality, caught up in a nightmare in which I could not distinguish myself from my surroundings."

Claustrophobia

The fear of closed places.

"We were on vacation when it first happened," explains a prominent businessman. "We had just gotten on a sight-seeing bus when I felt an overwhelming need to get off. I felt trapped, like I couldn't breathe. I knew I would suffocate if I didn't get back outside into the fresh air."

Another executive confesses, "I got into a car with some co-workers, and suddenly I was terrified that I was going to be ill. I sat near the window and kept thinking that I should jump out at the next stop, but I was too embarrassed. I was sure something awful was going to happen. I tried calculating how badly I'd be injured if I threw myself out while the car was still moving. Somehow I made it to work, but it was dreadful."

Depression and Frustration

Knowing the disease is persistent and out of control results in feelings of intense frustration.

One patient said, "My husband took my son out on a Sunday. It was a beautiful spring day, the kind that should be joyous. I wanted to go too, but I was afraid. I wanted to cry, just thinking about what I was missing, but I held back the tears so little Tim couldn't see.

When they drove off, I broke down and wept. I felt so sad that I crawled into bed and pulled the covers over my head; I wanted to die."

Avoidance

More and more activities are avoided so as not to trigger the dreaded attacks. Agoraphobics not only fear being outside, but as time passes, many things in their inside environment can become triggers, such as a fear of spiders.

"I always glance around any room I enter to see if there are spiders. I avoid cupboards, closets, corners, and dark places. I examine every bit of my salad to be sure a spider isn't hiding in the lettuce. Sometimes I even avoid salads altogether. I also stay clear of plants that might have spiders on them."

OTHER SYMPTOMS OFTEN EXPERIENCED BY AGORAPHOBICS

1.	Fatigue	7.	Irritability
2.	Tension	8.	Headaches
3.	Obsessive thoughts	9.	Palpitations
4.	Depression	10.	Fear of dying
5.	Loneliness	11.	Suicidal ideas
6.	Fear of fainting	12.	Fear of other diseases

Calamity Syndrome

Agoraphobia seldom begins in childhood. It usually emerges in women between the years of eighteen and thirty-five, often after a major physical or emotional ordeal. Agoraphobia has been called the "calamity syndrome" because the average patient suffers with it for over a decade, and many are never free of it.

It's difficult to say exactly how many people are afflicted with this disorder. It could be one out of every twenty or one out of ten; no one knows for sure because so many cases go undiagnosed. Many agoraphobics turn to liquor for relief, and get diagnosed as alcoholics, but they are really drinking to escape their panic. Many of the milder cases go unreported because the victims are housewives who stay at home and avoid treatment.

Although there is some evidence that the disease is hereditary, most patients are females from stable families with no history of behavioral problems. Prior to agoraphobia's onset, most of these patients have been described as shy, soft, passive, anxious, and dependent. But here again, there is no firm rule—many patients have been anxiety-free extroverts, with no signs of dependency. Nor do occupation and education seem to play a role in determining who will and who will not become agoraphobic. As with many diseases, it is no respecter of social class.

Agoraphobia should not be confused with social phobias where unreasonable anxiety is experienced in social situations and increases according to the size and formality of the occasion. (See Chapter 9 for an explanation of social phobias, and p. 169 for a list of symptoms of both agoraphobia and social phobias.) More men than women suffer from a social phobia, which is not as insidious as agoraphobia, because those who have one seldom suffer from multiple phobias.

Family Problems

The family inevitably becomes involved in agoraphobia; but because more women than men are victims, economic pressures are often not a factor when the husband is the primary breadwinner. Emotionally, however, the husband and other family members suffer significantly. The spouse and the children take over the burden of shopping and running errands and often must escort the patient whenever she goes out. Naturally, social activities become severely restricted. For some patients, the constant need for reassurance and companionship is so overwhelming that it becomes oppressive to their loved ones.

Conditions can become worse still if the agoraphobic consciously uses the illness for secondary gain. In some cases, a patient will manipulate family members at whim. If this pattern becomes apparent to the others, resentment and anger result and tension mounts. When the agoraphobic uses such tactics to attain selfish goals, she becomes unsure whether the others are acquiescing because they really care about her or merely because she has manipulated them. This increases the need for more reassurance, which in turn escalates tensions even further, all of which perpetuates a vicious and destructive cycle.

Stopping Phobias Before They Develop

We know that phobias often develop following a sudden trauma, although there is a certain period before it becomes apparent. Animal experiments suggest that immediate reexposure to the original situation during this lag phase may protect one against the development of future fears. Common lore has been to get people "back on the horse"—back into the pretraumatic situation immediately after the original trauma.

TREATING AGORAPHOBIA AND PANIC

The underlying causes of panic and agoraphobia are physical. We have already discussed the chemical abnormalities known to exist in panic patients. Fortunately, these chemical imbalances are not in play constantly but tend to fluctuate. Our goal then is not only to treat the physical causes but also to identify and stop the "triggers" that tip the scales out of balance. I have listed these triggers in Chapter 3, but I will quickly review them here as they relate to agoraphobia.

Food Allergies

Agoraphobics are frequently allergic to some foods that can trigger episodes of panic. To determine what your allergies are and deal with them, use the testing techniques in Chapter 3 and the treatment techniques mentioned in Chapter 4. If your food allergies are not clearly identified first, you may never have enough mental stability to conquer your problems. A patient of mine was found, like many others, to be allergic to some of her favorite foods. For example, oatmeal, her favorite breakfast dish, made her "spacey." Wheat made her panicky, and corn made her tired and irritable. If a patient, eating these foods daily, is constantly experiencing spaciness, fatigue, and irritability and is always on the verge of panic, it's easy to see how she would continually be fearful or suffer from anticipatory anxiety. Such a mental state is hardly conducive to successful treatment.

Chemical Allergies

Chemicals can also trigger anxiety and/or panic. Review Chapter 4 and deal with any chemical sensitivities that you suspect you may have. Avoid those chemicals that you know irritate you, and use nutritional supplements to neutralize those you can't avoid.

Hormone Imbalances

Premenstrual syndrome, menopause, or any other hormonal imbalances caused by the menstrual cycle may severely disturb the mental stability of female patients. Suggestions for dealing with this problem can be found in Chapter 7, but it's best to ask your family doctor for help. Menopausal symptoms are easily treated, and so is premenstrual syndrome. Hyperthyroidism is another imbalance frequently related to panic.

Physical Health

Your general physical condition has a bearing on the occurrence of panic attacks. As mentioned earlier, even such simple problems as anemia can trigger them. Chronic pollen allergies can tax your immune system as well as the nervous system, making you much more susceptible to anxiety and panic. And don't overlook the strain on your physical health that results from overwork. Review your priorities if you find yourself pushing too hard.

Energy

Motivation to accomplish anything requires energy. You can't fight a problem successfully if you don't have the staying power to follow through. The nutritional supplements that I recommend should be of great help, but you may need more. For example, if you experience muscle weakness or tire easily during the day, especially after work, you might need one or two 500 mg potassium tablets around 10 A.M. and again at 4 P.M. Whatever the reason for your lack of energy, do seek help for it. A good nutritionist or nutrition-minded physician can assist you.

Your Personal Relationships

If your life is a mess or you are just not getting along with others, it's important to pay some attention to this problem. If by making adjustments you can improve your personal life, then do so now, and take the strain off your anxiety system. If you're having difficulty doing this on your own, then see a counselor.

Therapy

Agoraphobia is such a severe disease that self-help is only a partial solution in nearly all cases. If you don't already have a counselor or a physician, you should definitely find one. The material in this book is meant to augment therapy, not replace it. It's also useful to have a support group. There are listings for these groups in Chapter 18, or you may find them in your telephone directory. If your therapist is acquainted with nutritional approaches, you may benefit even more.

Drugs

Avoid substances that are known to play havoc with mental stability (caffeine, sugar, cigarettes, alcohol, and recreational drugs). If necessary, get help to break these addictions. The chemicals in these substances act as panic triggers in most patients. Even prescription drugs may cause problems, especially medications, such as birth control pills, that affect hormones. Be aware of these hazards, and take appropriate precautions.

NUTRITIONAL TREATMENT

There are two approaches to nutritional treatment. The first is simply to use the nutritional supplements that have been found useful in the control of anxiety. This technique has the advantage of being less expensive to start with, but also has the disadvantage of not being as precise as a program based on diagnostic analysis. The second approach is to seek out a physician/nutritionist who does vitamin, mineral, and amino-acid analysis so that your exact blood and urine imbalances are identified.

The First Approach—Nutrients That Are Known to Work

1. Thiamine is always useful in calming anxiety. I usually start patients on one 500 mg tablet three times daily. This dosage may be increased or decreased, depending on the patient's response. Garlic oil capsules or liquid are also helpful—take twelve daily to start. This dosage can gradually be reduced as your symptoms decline.

2. Niacinamide is very important. I use 200 to 500 mg of niacinamide three times daily because of its relaxing effect.

3. Vitamin B_6 is crucial in making all of the amino acids work properly. Most people who are having problems with panic do not easily utilize B_6. A better form is paradoxyl-5-phosphate, 50 mg three or four times daily.

4. A good moderately strong multivitamin, mineral, and amino acid tablet should also be used. I recommend Nutra-Homo, one teaspoon of powder twice daily.

5. B_4, choline, is extremely important. Take one 1,000 mg tablet three times daily.

6. Calcium lactate has also been useful for relaxation response. I suggest one or two 500 mg tablets three times daily.

7. GABA is an amino acid that has been used with success, although in some unbalanced individuals it produces strong side effects. Obviously the start-up dosage should be low. I recommend one 500 mg tablet or ⅛ teaspoonful three times daily. Increase gradually to a quarter teaspoonful three times a day.

8. Ammonium chloride tablets, 7½ grams, have been found to assist GABA powder. Some patients find these helpful; others do not.

9. Tryptophan has been suggested and reported effective in treating panic and anxiety, although I have found it not to be as beneficial as others. Try one to three 500 mg tablets, three times daily.

10. A complete amino-acid capsule (containing all twenty-two amino acids) in addition to individual amino acids will balance individual amino acids which must be used in large amounts.

The Second Approach—Medical Analysis

In my office I usually do a blood and urine analysis for amino acids. Sometimes I also test for blood vitamins and minerals. Usually the results indicate gross disturbances in nutritional balances. All of the twenty-two amino acids are identified, making it easy to see what needs to be done. After a program is begun, we generally see dramatic results within several weeks. Consult the reference list of physicians in Chapter 18 for a doctor near you. This analysis must be done through a physician but is usually quick and successful.

Nutritional supplements definitely benefit agoraphobics, whether the relief is partial or complete. This approach is actually by far the most successful. All patients I have seen have responded to some degree, and most have been helped greatly. Some agoraphobics have needed to continue a little medication, but were able to take much less than before.

Nutritional and Psychological Treatment

Even though we are able to relieve panic completely, it is still necessary to *grow stronger* psychologically. That means you must still learn to face your fears even though you may not be suffering as you once did. You must go out, see people, do things, behave as normally as possible. You will need to stay on the nutritional supplements for at least a year. You may wish to check your progress at three- or four-month intervals, but you definitely should not try to stop the supplements for at least six months. If you have been steadily facing your fears, and if you have been able to find a good nutritional balance, it is possible that eventually you will be able to do without the supplements. The important thing in the long run is to keep improving your nutritional balance so that you can control your anxieties and enjoy a normal and happy life. Just as diabetics and hypertensive patients must often accept being forever dependent upon medication, agoraphobics may need to use supplements for indeterminate periods of time. Agoraphobia is a chronic disease, a physical disability that may require long-term and scrupulous control, but the results are well worth the effort.

Anxiety reduction by any method (progressive relaxation, hypnosis, carbon-dioxide treatment, or anxiety-reducing drugs) does not exempt patients from the need to learn new coping skills. Nor does the use of nutritional supplements, which reduce panic and anxiety, interfere with psychological progress. In fact, such a recovery process may be accelerated when anxiety is abated enough by medication or supplements to allow the patient to undertake a program of relearning and retraining.

Nutritional supplements in many cases provide rapid relief of symptoms, and patients may take them indefinitely to avoid recurrence and to accelerate a permanent return to normalcy. Supplements that reduce anxiety can be used along with any of the psychological treatments that follow.

PSYCHOLOGICAL METHODS TO HANDLE PANIC

If you have panic attacks or periods when you are near panic, you need to know how to prepare yourself for attacks that come without warning. Below are several exercises that will help you be prepared for your next panic episode. Following these exercises is a list of suggestions for what to do during the actual attack. If you have used the nutritional supplements already listed, you may find your attacks much less intense or you may experience them only when you have forgotten to take your supplements.

Train Your Fears—An Exercise to Practice Coping Behavior at Home Before You Go Out

You may wish to practice coping tactics before you actually experience a real-life situation. Then you can decide which of these methods might work best for you.

THE "BURN OUT" EXERCISE

You'll need to find time for a ten- to twenty-minute "rehearsal" as often as you can. Sit in an armchair or recliner, or simply lie down, close your eyes, then think of the most terrifying place you could possibly be. Let the anxiety flood over you, then use whichever coping behavior you have chosen from the list below. Work with it for several minutes, then rest, and keep repeating the process until you feel you have thoroughly learned the procedure. *Take your nutritional supplements one hour before you start the exercises.*

1. Say to yourself, "I'm going mad—I'm babbling incoherently, running uncontrolled, then I'm in a straitjacket, imprisoned and given shock treatment." Keep going over these scenes until they become routine.

2. Create a story about a horrifying event, and when you're overwhelmed by a frightening thought, force yourself to ask, "And then what happens." Keep the story going as long as you experience anxiety. For example, if you feel that you're going to have a heart attack, imagine the sequence of events. "I'll fall down, and people will see that I need help. Someone will call the paramedics. Then I'll have to go to the hospital in an ambulance." Don't stop: "They discover that it's not a heart problem, but that I'm going crazy. I'll be taken to a mental hospital." And then? "They give me medications and therapy. I start to respond to the treatment." And finally, "I get well enough to come home." Just continue the story, one step at a time, until your anxiety subsides.

3. "The plane is crashing, everyone is dying. I'm dead, in a morgue. The worst has happened, but now it's all over. There is nothing more to fear." Keep repeating this scenario until it loses its power.

Using anxiety-provoking stories such as these, you can stir up as much fear as possible for the purpose of using your coping techniques. Four useful coping techniques are listed below. If your nutritional supplements are working, it may be difficult to arouse much, if any, anxiety. Nevertheless, continue through the process without anxiety: learning can take place even when you are calm. Simply pretend you have anxiety, much as an actor would, then use the coping techniques to control your reactions.

COPING TECHNIQUE 1—CREATE A PLEASANT SCENE

Make up a pleasant scene, one that totally relaxes you. For example, picture yourself lying in a hammock near a lovely meadow under a shady tree. A gentle breeze cools this bright spring day. Rock back and forth. You have no place to go and nothing to do except to enjoy it. Keep visualizing specific objects in the scene; try to stay in that place until the anxiety subsides or you have a solidly fixed scene in your mind.

COPING TECHNIQUE 2—PARADOXICAL INTENTION

This technique is presented in Chapter 4. Reread and study it. This is probably the most useful technique available. Try to master it.

COPING TECHNIQUE 3—CHANGE YOUR TAPES

Since, as a patient, you may not initially be able to understand or explain the intense physiological responses you are experiencing, you may tend to invent your own answers. During your first or second panic attack, you probably decided, "I'm having a heart attack"; or "I'm going crazy." Although neither of those catastrophes becomes a reality, it may still cause you concern.

Step 1 Make up a list of all of the usual things you tell yourself during this time period, such as:

"I'm going to die!"
"They will take me away!"
"I'm going crazy!"
"I'm going to faint!"
"I must escape!"
"I've got to get out of here!"

Step 2 Before going out, rehearse each possibility. Reprogram your thinking and personal dialogues.

- "I can't handle shopping malls." Of course you can. "I'll be able to cope with the situation even if I'm uncomfortable and not relaxed."
- "I can't stand this anxiety!" Change that thought to "I may be anxious, but I can cope with physical discomfort."
- "I'll never be able to stay in this situation." Yes, you will. "I'm not in any danger; I'm just feeling uncomfortable for a while. It's not pleasant, but it isn't the worst feeling I've ever had in my life, and it's helping me get over my fears so that the next time won't be so bad."
- "I'll lose my mind, or I'll completely fall apart if I stay here." That won't happen. "I have been through this before, and I've never gone crazy. I can do it again, even though I may feel overwhelmed. I'm staying in control. I'll be able to manage regardless of what happens. I'll do this by concentrating on the business at hand, such as shopping, driving, etc."
- "My heart is pounding; I'm going to have a coronary!" Instead, tell yourself, "My body is merely behaving as though I were running a race. My signals are a bit confused."
- "I feel as though I might faint and embarrass myself." What if you do? "I'm not going to pass out. Agoraphobics don't actually faint, they just feel as though they might."
- "I could embarrass myself by acting crazy." So what? "These people don't know what I'm feeling. They are so involved in their own lives they're not paying much attention. If they did know what I'm going through, they'd probably be sympathetic." Continue on and take charge of every thought, then change it to a positive affirmation.

COPING TECHNIQUE 4—THE WRITTEN MESSAGE

Although this technique may seem simplistic, it has proved effective for some people. All you need is to write reassuring messages in a notebook or diary and throughout the day constantly repeat them.

"I will be all right."

"No matter what happens, I will survive."

At the First Sign of a Real Anxiety Attack, Use Your "Tricks"

When you first experience a fear, take action. At the onset of anxiety, use one of your "tricks" to control it. The more intense your feelings are before you exert control, the harder they are to deal with. Try to recognize the first signs of panic and act immediately. A funny sensation in the stomach, a tingling in the skin, an unexplained premonition, a slight dizziness—any minor signs of an impending anxiety attack—that's the moment to move into action.

Learn to understand your fears. A panic or anxiety attack is the result of a disturbed body chemistry and nervous system. Your body has become disorganized, and all the signal lights on the switchboard are flashing. Fighting it, or trying to run away, only worsens the situation. When the attack occurs, concentrate on remaining where you are until your body has time to become acclimated. Remember that the body in its own wisdom is trying to reorganize the signals gone awry, and it will do so on its own if you stay calm and use the proper techniques. Giving in to your feelings and fully experiencing them is an effective way of helping your body gain control.

But how long can you endure such discomfort? In most cases, an anxiety attack which is not made worse by incorrect reactions will last (at the most) twenty or thirty minutes, then it will begin to subside and should be over completely in about an hour.

If you happen to be in a market, for example, you might try remaining in one spot, pretending that you're reading the ingredients on a can. Or you can quickly go to your car and sit down and wait for your body to return to normal. Rate your fears on a scale of one to a hundred, and watch the clock. Use any of the tricks you've learned to get through the worst part. You can and should go ahead with your daily activities even with residual tension, for continuing to function will increase your confidence and hasten recovery.

If an Attack Occurs, There Are Many Ways to Cope

1. Say to yourself the things you've practiced in the "burn out" exercise.

2.   Distract yourself. Count the number of windows in a building. Count the books or boxes on a shelf. Keep searching for things to keep your mind busy. All you have to do is kill some time until the panic subsides.

3.   Slow down your breathing, take deep breaths, feel the temperature of the air in your nose and lungs. Get in touch with your chest muscles.

4.   Go from head to toe on your body systematically and tighten and relax various muscle groups. Do it slowly, one at a time. Use any muscle relaxation technique you know.

5.   Close your eyes and get in touch with sounds around you. Traffic, people talking, air conditioners, airplanes, etc.

6.   Getting mad as hell at anything can help break up panic, but the anger must be real and intense.

7.   Turn to prayer. Recite the Lord's Prayer. Use religious bead counting. Whatever works.

8.   Memorize words or phrases and repeat them endlessly almost as if you were chanting, but listen to their meaning at the same time.

9.   Count backwards from 100, by threes.

10.   Physically touch anyone or anything around you often or continuously. You might hold hands or make physical contact with others.

11.   If you should think negative thoughts, such as "I wonder what others are thinking of me," be aggressive with yourself. Say, "To hell with what they think!" Panic attacks are embarrassing and upsetting, but that is all. You have no more reason to be ashamed than someone who suffers from migraines or ulcers.

After You Are Back at Home, Give Yourself a Pat on the Back

1.   "I did very well, considering."

2.   "I did pretty well."

3. "I didn't let my nervousness completely control me."
4. "I realize that I really have more control over this than I thought."
5. "I am proud of the way I stayed at the mall in spite of my anxiety."
6. "I'm pleased with myself for not running away and letting my fears get the best of me."

If You Are Invited to a Party—Accept the Invitation, Then Make Your Plans

1. Preplan an excuse, in case you need to leave, such as getting up early the next day, or caring for a sick child.

2. Don't drink alcohol or eat the sweets at the party. Take three 500 mg L-glutamine tablets with two chromium tablets to stop cravings. Panic attacks are often set off by sugar and alcohol. Of course, don't eat any foods you are allergic to.

3. Go to the party hoping to have a panic attack so that you can practice managing it.

4. Face up to the worst that can happen, then get up and go to the party.

5. The worst thing that can happen is embarrassment, and you can live with that.

6. The next worst thing is the feeling that you have lost control over your body and mind, but you are putting an end to that by seeking out the problem on your own terms.

7. Go with a friend.

8. Take your regular nutritional supplements before you go and take a second dose that you can use halfway through the party.

Training Away the Fears by Facing Them Gradually

This method is called desensitization. The technique is as old as the hills, but it has proven to be a reliable and useful way to get rid of fears. It is being used successfully by clinics around the country, and although sometimes slow and cumbersome, this self-help method may be the right approach for some readers. If it appeals to you, use it. If not, go on to other techniques.

You may gradually face your feared object or situation through imagery or you can do it in real life. I will explain the "mental" and then the "real-life" approach. If you're apprehensive, try the self-imagery first.

Take your nutritional supplements a half hour before each session, and you may sail right through these exercises. Remember that you must repeatedly expose yourself to your phobias, with or without anxiety. Just because you can face your fears with nutritional supplements does not mean you could easily do so without them. The point of this treatment is to expose yourself to your fears often enough so that you can face them without the supplements, and without discomfort.

Desensitization—Practice at Home

Phobias are partially learned. To eliminate unnecessary anxiety and fear, you must re-create the original learning experience or something similar without the accompanying pain. While reexperiencing a particular trauma, the patient can learn to extinguish the anxiety that supports his pathological system of behavior.

First make a list of ten situations leading up to the most fearful situation you can imagine. Begin with the least fearful event and end with the one that causes you the most distress. To determine just how fearful each situation is, consider an imaginary scale of one to ten, with one being no fear at all, and ten representing absolute terror. Two and three would be mild fear, four to six moderate fear, seven strong fear, eight and nine near panic and full panic. Ten is unmitigated terror. Now, rate each of the situations you have listed. In making your ranking, omit any scenes that don't make you respond at least to the point of five. Skip all items below that point.

Get into a comfortable chair in a quiet room with the lights dimmed. Close your eyes, relax, and clear your mind. Work with the first image you have listed. Run it through your mind over and over so that it becomes less and less frightening. Stay with it as long as you can tolerate the attendant anxiety. A session should usually last twenty to thirty minutes; and under normal circumstances, most people will only get through one or two items on their list at one time. You may stop if you feel you need to, but on the other hand, you should try to progress as quickly as possible. Often those using nutritional supplements prior to imaging can get through five to eight steps in one session. It is important that you make every attempt to create the situations as vividly as possible. Use your imagination to the best of your ability, and see, hear, feel, touch, and smell everything in the scene that you possibly can.

Don't continue to the next fearful image on your list unless you have brought your fears down to at least a one or zero. Keep repeating the scene until you get a zero or one at least twice. Do not worry about the order of presentations. Studies have shown good results no matter what order they occur in. You may find it a little easier, however, to tackle the least frightening scenes first, but if you feel brave, then start at the top. Just be sure you have really vanquished each anxiety before moving on. If the next step is too upsetting, then drop back and repeat each one until you can do them at least twice without anxiety.

How many sessions does it take to train yourself out of your fears? That depends on the individual. In therapy, patients usually hold their sessions twice weekly for six to twelve weeks. You may do them, however, as often as you wish.

If you find yourself quickly able to face your most frightening situation, then just go straight to that one at the beginning of each session. You may then want to create several more, equally fearful situations to add to your repertoire. It usually takes anywhere from a week to one month to establish controllable fear levels in phobic situations.

Desensitization—Away from Home

1.   Spend an hour developing a list of gradually more adventurous outings to be carried out at your own pace.

2.   Agoraphobics should make a list of all the places and things normally avoided. Then select the four main target phobias to be faced; for example, walking alone, supermarkets, business situations, airplanes.

3. Rank each activity by the intensity of your fear—one, two, three, etc.

4. Decide on a specific time and place to face your first targeted phobia. You may wish to be accompanied by a friend on the first three outings.

5. Set up sessions of one hour or more twice a week for two weeks, then once a week for four weeks. You may schedule them a lot more frequently than this if you wish.

6. Take no sugar, alcohol, or stimulants for six hours prior to the treatment, and, if possible, refrain entirely on the day of the treatments. That includes having no tea, coffee, diet colas, or recreational drugs.

7. Take your nutritional formula 45 minutes before starting the treatment.

8. Make your transportation arrangements in advance, and be sure to leave on time.

9. Go to the intimidating area or as close to it as you can, and remain there as long as possible.

10. If you were not able to reach your phobic spot, but stopped short, you might find that after waiting a while, your anxiety diminishes or ceases altogether. Remember that you're supposed to allow a full hour in which to face your fears.

EXAMPLE OF FEAR OF LEAVING HOME

First decide where you're going to go. Are you going to walk or drive? Let's suppose you have decided to walk to a nearby market five blocks away. You may wish to walk alone, or you may ask a friend to meet you there and accompany you home. That is enough for your first day out. On the next trip you may go to a nearby department store, leaving your friend outside while you spend some time in the store. Later, you may want to use public transportation with or without a friend. As you can see, the object is to get farther and farther away from home and to take more and more risks. One patient of mine used a bicycle and pedaled farther away from home each day.

Usually the nutritional supplements will protect you from panic, and you will find yourself easily able to go where you please. But just because you now are free to go doesn't mean the job is over. For your own well-being and personal growth, it is necessary that you face your fears. So continue with the program. Test yourself frequently to see how your fear levels are changing. A diary would be of great benefit.

If you return from an excursion and feel anxious, take a warm bath and relax with the satisfaction that you have faced the same exhausting emotions as a mountain climber. Congratulate yourself on your courage and achievement. You have just completed a very difficult task. Give yourself a pat on the back for trying.

Don't forget to use the valuable coping techniques listed in Chapter 4. Review the section on Paradoxical Intention; as an assist to the nutritional supplements, it is tremendously helpful, for it can reduce tensions in a matter of seconds.

SUMMARY OF DESENSITIZATION METHOD

1.   Fears are a physical phenomenon, a disturbance of the signaling system which tells your body that you're in danger. This false call-up of the body's defenses can cause discomfort and anxiety, but disturbed signals do not mean that your body is being harmed.

2.   Fears tend to dissipate with time. The longer you can force yourself to tolerate an unpleasant anxiety, the sooner it will subside.

3.   Facing your worst situations first will hasten your speed of recovery. Taking it too "easy" will only stretch out the time it takes to get well.

4.   If you feel you must go slowly, list all of the situations you have difficulty with and rate them—relatively easy, very difficult, and nearly impossible.

Start with the easy ones first, then pick one and do it. Use your chosen technique to fight each fear, and stay with it for an hour and even longer if possible. Keep repeating the process until you are no longer afraid. When you have conquered the relatively easy ones, proceed to anxieties that are more difficult to face.

Use a Helper

Nonprofessional former phobics make excellent therapists. People who have already dealt successfully with their own symptoms can be very effective helpers because they are aware of all the problems and have plenty of empathy with other agoraphobics (Ross 1980). It is an inspiration to be with those who have "made it," and it's valuable to spend time discussing what they went through and how they achieved success. A phobic support group meeting might be a good starting place to locate such a helper—or you might even try advertising in the paper. A good friend could also be supportive if he or she is someone who would understand and be noncritical. But if necessary, you can do the job yourself.

THE RUNNING TREATMENT

This treatment for agoraphobia needs to be used more often, but it is quite effective. If you fancy yourself a jogger or would like to add fitness to your method of overcoming your fears, then consider this method.

Before You Run

- Prepare a set of destinations close enough to walk or run to from your house. Each destination should be about as far as you can go without experiencing overwhelming panic. Your first outing might cover half a block, or up to several blocks. The second might be six to eight blocks, and after that, you can continue to extend the distance at a comfortable pace.
- Make an estimate of how far you can run before getting winded. Let's say, for our purposes, that would be about one city block.
- Take your nutritional supplements an hour before you run.
- Just before you leave, take one 500 mg potassium tablet, one

or two 400-unit vitamin E capsules, and if possible, eat one salted, soft-boiled egg; a salted, hard-boiled egg is the next choice.

- Now decide whether you want to run or walk fast. The choice is yours, so do whatever is more comfortable.

FAST WALK

1. Make an estimate of how far you think you can walk before running out of steam. You must be walking as fast as possible. (Example: two city blocks.)

2. Your first day out, determine your initial destination. If it is less than two blocks from your house, walk in place until you get tired, then walk away from home until you are completely out of breath or until your anxiety becomes great. You can always take a bus back and conveniently sit or stand unnoticed behind others.

3. Second destination: Let's say it's four blocks away. Walk at a normal pace for two blocks, then walk fast for two more blocks, until you arrive breathless at your destination. If you feel you could go farther, continue on until you are forced to stop either by fatigue or anxiety. Stay out as long as you can, then return home.

RUNNING

1. Estimate how far you can run before tiring. (Example: one city block.)

2. First day: If your destination is one block or less, then begin running when you leave your house and stop when you are out of breath or have too much anxiety. Rest a while, then return home.

3. Second destination: Let's say it's four blocks away. Walk normally for three blocks, then run one block so you arrive at your destination out-of-breath. If you think you can continue past this point, do so until you are compelled to stop because of breathlessness or anxiety. Stay there as long as you can, then return home.

4. Continue adding to the distance you go, increasing two blocks each time, until you reach your walking limits. Always start your fast walk two blocks before your new destination.

4. Continue extending your distance until you can't go any farther. Always run the last block.

Variations for Running Treatment

If you know your neighborhood well or if you study a map, you can envision a circle around your house. You will find a series of streets that will always keep you about the same distance from home. Following one of these routes, run a circle around your house, always staying about the same number of blocks away. Always walk fast or run the last block or two. Your second circle would always keep you, let's say, four blocks away from home.

It is not necessary to run or fast-walk the complete circle. You can always stop and rest any time or place you wish. The important thing is to stay out for as long as you feel is tolerable. And when I say tolerable, I don't mean comfortable. I'm talking about the highest levels of anxiety you can handle and still feel in control. When you think you are going to actually lose control, then return home.

- If you have any health problems or you're unsure of your physical condition, consult a physician before starting these jaunts.
- You may do this daily, or twice a day or once a week. You may create your own treatment schedule in advance or make it up as you go along. Let your body and your mind tell you what the best pace would be.
- If you feel yourself burning out or becoming overwhelmed by the sessions, rest a few days, then start again at a slower pace. If you feel you're progressing rapidly, and you have the time and spirit, increase the number of sessions.

How long before you'll get any benefits? That depends on a number of factors. Mild cases usually become symptom free in ten to fifteen sessions. Moderate cases often are free of agoraphobia symptoms in twenty to thirty sessions. Severe cases might take thirty to ninety times out. If you use nutritional supplements, these figures can be reduced considerably.

All this may seem like a lot of work. But patients with agoraphobia can be incapacitated for twenty to thirty years. A therapy that leads to the reversal of years of unhappiness can't be too high a price to pay, even when the going is tough. And as side benefits, you'll improve your cardiovascular system, and perhaps even lose a few pounds.

Dress for All Occasions

Get into the habit of wearing jogging suits when you go to the market or out shopping. For a while, try to shop in small centers near a residential area rather than in central city locations. That way, if a panic attack occurs, simply go outside and fast-walk or jog until you are breathless.

THE FIVE-MINUTE PHOBIA CURE

In 1985, Dr. Roger J. Callahan, Ph.D., wrote an interesting book called *The 5-Minute Phobia Cure* (Enterprise Publishing Inc., 1985). He suggests the use of a technique called applied kinesiology. This is a method used mostly by chiropractors, based on the theory that there are meridians at different locations on the surface of the body identical or similar to Chinese acupuncture points. Certain spots on these meridians, if tapped, produce a permanent phobia cure, according to Callahan, who claims an 85 percent success rate using this technique. I suggest you read his book, if you are interested in learning how to use the method correctly. Treatment involves using your index finger to press carefully on the bony spot directly below the center of the eye nearest the lower eyelid. Press both sides carefully for thirty seconds while clearly imagining the subject of your phobia. Next, for thirty seconds, tap on the outside of each of your second toes (next to the big toe), while visualizing a fearful situation.

Dr. Callahan has a number of routines to follow if the first one does not work. I have talked to some patients who have used his techniques, and most said they helped to some degree but did not relieve their fears completely. This method might be another good weapon to add to your stockpile, since anything that brings about improvement is worthwhile.

I would advise you, however, to use a nutritional routine for several weeks before beginning this treatment.

Summary

Nutritional supplements can be used to eliminate or at least considerably reduce all fears. Keep working with the supplements until you have arrived at a comfortable state. Nutritional supplements are excellent for controlling anxiety; but, in order to complete the job, it is necessary to do some personal growing. That means facing your fears, using the recommended methods.

In this chapter, you have been given the basic ideas for creating your own nutritional program, and various psychological methods for dealing with and conquering your fears. Does that mean someday you may be able to stop the supplements? For many patients, the answer is yes; for a few, the answer is no; and for others, the answer lies somewhere in between. Heredity, attitude, and your willingness to grow affect the outcome.

6

How to Conquer the Panic and Fears Related to Alcoholism

"Don't you ever take a drink again. *Do you hear me?* ... Take a look at yourself. You're jaundiced. Your skin is yellow because your liver is totally shot. Do you hear me?" Dr. Johnson's stubby fat finger flashed under Judy's nose like a signal at a railroad crossing. "If you ever take a drink again, you're going to *die*. Do you want to die?" he demanded. Not waiting for an answer, he continued, "Are you listening to me?"

The voice trailed off in Judy's head. Her mind was swirling. Her wires were shorting out. She was beyond crying; she was shattering into fragments like pottery, falling into dust on her hospital bed. Judy's brain screamed, "I can't take this. I'm just over the DTs and now this. Why did they bring me to the hospital? Why not just let me die at home?" *"You won't live for a week,"* the harangue sliced through her thoughts again. Please, Dr. Johnson, please, she silently pleaded for him to stop. Panic gripped her heart, and her mind raced off in all directions, trying to make sense out of the unconnected phrases. She looked at the doctor through a veil of tears.

"Take one more drink and you've had it, kid" was his parting shot as he closed the door to the hospital room behind him, sending a gust of cold air to chill Judy's body in its sweat-soaked hospital gown. She was a pathetic, lonely figure, trapped in a strange and horrible place. A few minutes later the walls began to close in on her. . . .

I was at the nurses' station ten days later when I overheard some patients talking about Judy. She had just been found dead in her apartment after an intense bout of drinking. From what I could piece together, she had checked herself out of the hospital the day after Dr. Johnson berated her and, in a terrible panic, did what she always did when frightened—she sought refuge in the bottle.

Dr. Johnson, attempting to scare her into changing her way of life, had produced in Judy the very emotion that compelled her to drink—fear. And Judy predictably responded as she always did, by getting drunk. She had to get rid of her fears the quickest way she knew how, the *only* way she knew how to cope. If Dr. Johnson had been aware that fear was Judy's problem, he might have abandoned his moralistic, self-righteous attitude and tried to understand the dynamics that were destroying his patient. He could have tried to keep her anxiety under control until some sort of therapy had been initiated. Unfortunately, his naive approach proved deadly.

Anxiety and fear play a crucial role in drinking behavior in certain alcoholics. The purpose of this chapter is to focus on such people and to suggest nutritional supplements that may help them control the anxiety and fears which contribute to their alcoholism.

I believe that although all alcoholics may benefit from the nutritional supplements listed in this chapter, they are especially useful for that one third of the general alcoholic population whose incapacitating fears and anxieties cause their excessive drinking. A second third, who sometimes drink in response to fear and anxiety and whose phobias are on an intermediate level, will also receive help.

First and foremost, it should be understood that no single treatment, including nutritional supplements, should be the *only* method of treating alcoholism. It is an extremely tenacious disease, and an alcoholic determined to cure his addiction needs *all* the help he can get. The supplements suggested here are meant primarily to reduce panic and phobias that cause certain alcoholics to drink. With this pressure removed, they will be more able to respond to other methods of treatment. If these supplements are used properly, many alcoholics in this group may not require any medication at all. If medication is necessary, it may be prescribed in substantially smaller doses than usual.

THE IMPORTANCE OF CLASSIFYING ALCOHOLICS

Developing patient profiles and laboratory tests to better identify the underlying causes and triggers of alcoholism is an essential step toward implementing more specific treatments. This is critically important when you consider that approximately 85 percent of all alcoholics never undergo treatment, and over 75 percent of those who do receive help fail to overcome their abuse of alcohol.

It may surprise you to learn that there has never been a serious, concentrated effort to separate the different causal factors that are responsible for alcoholism. In other areas of medicine, virtually all treatments are based on cause. As we know, headaches are not all alike; some are due to tension, others result from sinusitis or allergy, and a few may be symptomatic of a brain tumor. Obviously, the treatment for each type of headache is different. Do not make the mistake of assuming that all causes of alcoholism are fully recognized and understood. *They are not.* A search of the medical literature quickly reveals that researchers are still seeking answers, and they are nowhere near any definite conclusions.

The American Psychiatric Association has divided alcoholism into only two general categories: psychological addiction and physiological addiction. The tendency is to identify more and more cases as biochemically based. Is this a correct interpretation? In his work *The Disease Concept of Alcoholism*, Jellineck divided types of alcoholism into two groups: gamma and delta. A gamma alcoholic most often complains of a loss of self-control. He is unable to stop drinking once he begins. A delta alcoholic, on the other hand, indulges in binge drinking. Jellineck also defined a fluid group of "non-addictive" alcoholics, who had suffered health problems but were not classically addicted. These groups were presented merely as rough classifications upon which to base further study. These two examples reveal how simplistic the efforts have been so far. Researchers in the area of alcoholism have long been critical of this scientific shortcoming.

Most treatment facilities do not attempt to subclassify their patients with regard to the cause of their alcoholism. As a result, their generalized treatment plan usually consists of confining the alcoholic to a mental health unit for a short period of intensive therapy.

Outpatient treatment usually follows, including some individual counseling and/or group therapy where patients can ventilate their feelings.

How useful is such treatment? A 1976 study by J. Orford and G. Edwards showed no statistical difference between the recovery rates of treated and untreated alcoholics. Other studies show that 20 to 30 percent of all untreated alcoholics may manage to control their addiction for twelve months, which is the same success rate as those who undergo treatment. The actual benefit received by alcoholics in present, orthodox, medical management programs is highly questionable. In fact, some researchers have gone so far as to say that the present medical approach to alcoholism is totally ineffective except for initial detoxification.

Why am I making such a point of this need for solid classification within the disease? Because this book offers a viable solution to one group of alcoholics who drink primarily because of their compelling need to quell their anxiety and phobias. This group, if identified and treated correctly, has an excellent chance of being successfully helped. Evidence verifies that in a high percentage of these cases, when panic attacks and phobias are controlled, so is the alcoholism.

J. A. Mullaney and C. J. Trippet report in their research summary that a third of the 102 alcoholics in their treatment unit suffered from crippling cases of agoraphobia or social phobia that had existed before they were diagnosed as alcoholics. Another third had the same problems to a lesser degree, and a final third were free of such symptoms. The problems seemed to appear during the teenage years or early twenties. In general, there were more males than females who turned to alcohol for relief from tension. It may also be noted that the percentage of alcoholics found to be phobic is much larger than that of the general population, and the milder the phobias, the later the alcoholism tends to develop.

Authors of a number of recent medical papers ask clinicians to be aware of the relationship between phobias and alcoholism, for if detected early enough, long-term physical and psychological deterioration can be prevented.

C. J. Hudson and S. H. Perkins have stated that alcoholics who insist on having a friend or relative accompany them to therapy, or always demand to sit near a door, should be suspected of being phobic. There are also a number of reliable psychological tests that can be used to diagnose such individuals.

Drugs for Anxiety and Panic in Alcoholics—Or Not?

Most doctors tend to write prescriptions for alcoholics, a practice strongly opposed by lay groups such as Alcoholics Anonymous. If the alcoholic is trying to stay dry and avoid panic and phobias at the same time, he or she has a *real* problem because the only present treatment for acute panic or anxiety is medication.

Another problem is the possibility of drug habituation which only complicates such therapy. A severe panic attack is an extremely distressing experience because of its unpredictability in social situations. The sheer dread of such an attack only increases the tension. If an alcoholic has given up the drinking once needed to calm him, then medication merely takes its place. Though imipramine and other antidepressants used to treat panic attacks are not addictive per se, a patient can eventually become psychologically dependent on them, posing a real dilemma for both physician and patient. This also raises the long-argued question of whether or not it is proper to prescribe mind-altering drugs to those who tend to abuse them in the first place.

NUTRITIONAL SUPPLEMENTATION TO CONTROL PANIC PHOBIAS AND THE CRAVINGS FOR ALCOHOL

Although Chapter 2 covers the following three nutrients in great detail because they stabilize that center of the brain that relates most to anxiety, let me summarize their benefits here because I suggest their use in the treatment of alcoholism.

Calcium is an essential neurochemical in the nerve conduction system. Without it, a person's nerves will become very sensitive, producing irritability, anxiousness, tension, and fear. Calcium is also essential to the biochemical conduction system within the cells. Every cell in the body requires adequate amounts of this mineral in order to initiate enzyme reactions. When calcium is not present in adequate amounts, general malaise results. Research also shows that blood and body tissues high in acid will tie up calcium, and when this happens, individuals will become anxious and have a panic attack. One 500 mg tablet three times a day.

Vitamin B$_1$ is important not only to normal nerve conduction but also in its relationship to fear levels. When individuals are deprived of B$_1$, in addition to other symptoms they develop panic attacks and chronic high fear levels. I have the patients take 500 mg tablets of B$_1$ three times daily in the beginning. Individuals in this category should reread Chapter 2 in order to make the variations necessary to reach the optimum level. Skip this if you use liver tablets, discussed below.

Choline is a vitamin that becomes a part of acetylcholine, a neurotransmitter known for its calming effect. The sympathetic nervous system discharges excessively during moments of panic and is opposed by the parasympathetic nervous system. Choline will help activate the parasympathetic system and thus calm a nervous individual. When taken in conjunction with B$_1$, it intensifies the vitamin's calming effect, thus giving the person additional benefit. I prescribe 1,000 mg of choline three times a day along with the B$_1$.

The following supplements have been used successfully in medical treatment clinics, so I recommend them to all of my patients who suffer from alcoholism.

1. *Evening primrose oil* can be specifically helpful to alcoholics. The best source, at the most reasonable cost, is a company called "Cardiovascular Research" in Oakland, California. The address is:

1061-B Sharry Circle
Concord, California
94518

Take four capsules each morning and four in the evening. Do not use substitutes because they won't provide the same effect. Health food store owners often tend to suggest alternative items if they don't carry a particular product, so don't be misdirected. Effects of evening primrose oil may take a few weeks or months to become noticeable, but it eventually diminishes the craving for alcohol and acts as a rejuvenating agent for the liver by improving detoxification in the body.

2. For the many alcoholics who have difficulty sleeping because the hypothalamus has been greatly traumatized by excess alcohol,

I recommend up to 4,000 mg of *tryptophan* at bedtime. Tablets in 500 mg doses can be purchased at any local health food store. This supplement has also proven to be helpful for suicide-prone alcoholics. Research has shown that depletion of the brain neurohormone serotonin is the most likely physiological cause of suicides, and alcohol causes its depletion. Tryptophan with a little honey at bedtime will replace the deficit, increase the restorative effect of sleep, and, in addition, will decrease overall depression. During the day 500 mg tryptophan tablets may also be used when needed to help relieve depression or anxiety. Taking 200 mg of niacinamide and one or two aspirins along with the tryptophan is helpful. A product called Tryptoplex by Tyson Labs is also good.

3.   *Liver tablets*, twelve 5-gram tablets taken throughout the day, will provide a good source of B vitamins along with the energy boost an alcoholic often needs. (If you are allergic to beef, do not use this supplement.)

4.   *Vitamin C* in powder form benefits alcoholics. Take 8,000 mg a day, half in the morning and half in the early evening. Most C powders come 4,000 mg to a teaspoonful, so use one teaspoonful in the morning and one in the evening.

5.   *Vitamin B_6* is necessary for alcoholics; taking 50 mg three times daily will supply energy and assist dozens of enzyme systems necessary for a healthy metabolism. (If your doctor advises you to take larger doses of B_6, be cautious, as it is believed to create cases of permanent nerve damage. More than 200 mg daily can be harmful.)

6.   *L-glutamine* is an energy-giving amino acid known to stop alcoholic cravings. More important, it functions as a GABA producer, a critical enzyme that blocks the runaway stimulatory effect of the emotional part of the brain. Take six 500 mg tablets of L-glutamine three times daily, and more as needed if a craving occurs. Since it is a food supplement, it is safe even in larger doses.

SUMMARY OF NUTRITION FOR ALCOHOLICS

1.   Evening primrose oil   4 capsules in the morning. 4 capsules in the evening.

2. Tryptophan, 500 mg tablets   8 at bedtime for sleep and 1 every 4 hours in the daytime if nervous.

3. Liver tablets, 5 gm   4 tablets 3 times daily, up to a total of 20 daily.

4. Vitamin C powder   8,000 mg a day, half in the morning and half in the evening.

5. Vitamin B_6, 50 mg tablets   1 tablet 3 times daily.

6. L-glutamine, 500 mg tablets   6 tablets 3 times daily, more if needed during the day to total of 20.

These are the suggested doses for the average adult, but they should be tailored to fit the needs of each individual. When these supplements are taken properly, side effects rarely occur. A balanced diet is vital to a recovering alcoholic. Food intake can affect cravings, energy levels, emotionalism, depression, concentration, memory, and coordination.

FOOD ALLERGIES: THE CAUSE OF ALCOHOLISM?

Alcoholism epitomizes the food addiction problem. The drink addict is not hooked on alcohol itself, but rather on one or more of the foods from which these beverages are derived.

When we discuss allergies, most people think of allergies to dust, pollens, and danders that cause sneezing or rashes. When we speak of food allergies, they think of strawberries causing hives. People are not yet aware that many food allergies go undetected because they cause symptoms we have never associated with our eating patterns. Foods can exert their allergic effect on the nervous system and can cause depression, irritability, anger, hyperactivity, fatigue, headaches, and a feeling of "spaciness." These symptoms and many others are discussed in Dr. Theron Randolph and R. W. Moss's book

An Alternative Approach to Allergies (Lippincott and Crowell, 1979). Our interest at the moment is in one profound symptom—the tendency toward cravings, specifically the craving for alcohol.

Allergy Addiction

This is a condition which causes an individual to crave the very thing to which he is allergic. The first effect of consuming the addictive food is an increase in metabolism, causing a "rush" of energy. The pulse accelerates and one feels instantly "better"; this is commonly referred to as a "high." After a while, the high wears off, but instead of returning to normal, the individual then suffers a drop in energy. He may become moody or irritable as he goes into withdrawal phase; now he is experiencing a "low." To get relief from this "low," he eats more of the food that made him feel good. The patient quickly discovers that, if he continuously eats food he is allergic to, he can "ride the highs" without having to come down. If for some reason he is deprived of that food, he will not feel well, and he will have an urgent craving for it. He is now fully addicted and doesn't feel "right" without his "fix." The reason why this vicious cycle is often ignored is that food is a necessity, and because it is nearly always available, the "foodaholic" need never develop full-blown withdrawal symptoms.

According to this theory, it is not the ethanol in alcohol that alcoholics crave but the other ingredients (foods), with which the alcohol has been mixed. In *An Alternative Approach to Allergies*, Dr. Randolph states that he discovered many of his alcoholic patients were allergic to corn, wheat, or yeast, all common ingredients in alcoholic beverages. He cites the case of a business executive who, because of out-of-control drinking, went from Wall Street to skid row.

The patient was finally able, with the help of his family, to remain sober for ten years, but then he began to backslide. At this point, Dr. Randolph started testing him for food allergies. When he ingested corn, the patient began to stagger as though he had suddenly become drunk. The next day he experienced a hangover as intense as those produced by heavy drinking. The doctor deduced that this man's cravings for alcohol were an attempt to avoid withdrawal symptoms by getting cereal grains into his system and thus perpetuating the stimulation provided by the allergy-producing food. By avoiding cereal grains, the patient eliminated his cravings for alcohol.

When food cravings are interpreted as an urgent need to drink, a hellish sort of merry-go-round begins for the alcoholic. If willpower is the only weapon, results are often unsuccessful, because an alcoholic who is allergic-addicted to cereal grains cannot eat *any* foods containing these items (bread, bakery products, breakfast cereals, etc.) without craving alcohol, since all of these foods serve as a trigger. The alcoholic can never be free from his problem as long as he consumes the foods that provoke his desire to drink.

Dr. Randolph also discovered that a patient, allergic-addicted to the sugar in alcohol, would sometimes carry a pocketful of candies to suck on whenever he had the urge to drink. This behavior apparently occurs when alcoholics instinctively learn to give themselves a little dose of what they crave, as a substitute for alcohol. The problem with using candy as a substitute for alcohol is that while it may provide some temporary relief, it endlessly perpetuates the desire for alcohol, and the cycle goes on.

If alcoholics are not physically addicted to ethyl alcohol, as was once thought, but are instead addicted to its food bases, then theoretically a patient may drink some types of beverages (such as certain rums and wines) without losing control. Unfortunately, all alcoholic beverages contain yeast, so if an alcoholic is yeast allergic, he must abstain altogether.

Diet

Caffeine is possibly the most abused of all substances because of its wide use. It is contained in coffee, tea, diet colas, and other soft drinks and will quickly deplete vitamins and stimulate the sympathetic nervous system, the very system you do *not* want stimulated.

Sugar and all forms of sweets should also be avoided. Sugar "primes the pump," as well as causing food allergy symptoms that may lead to hypoglycemia.

The first thing an alcoholic will often do is turn to soda pop or junk food, or fill his coffee cup with sugar. As a result, he or she may develop such hypoglycemic symptoms as depression, irritability, insomnia, weakness, fatigue, and anger. The inevitable next step is toward alcohol for relief. The best way to avoid this is to take L-glutamine four or five times a day with a little protein (a hard-boiled egg or a piece of chicken) and salt. Salt will relieve hypoglycemic symptoms as quickly and easily as sugar, though you may not have any craving for it. Also, beware of sweet fruit juices. They are often used as a substitute for candy under the guise of being "healthy," but in fact, a glass of orange juice contains slightly more sugar than many soft drinks. Vegetable juices, which are sugar free, are a safe and pleasurable alternative. During the worst stages of alcohol craving, you can increase your water intake to eight or ten glasses a day, but refrain from any other beverages. High fluid levels greatly diminish cravings.

Diversify your diet by eating simple, whole foods. Many people tend to eat a "mono" diet—the same thing day after day. Avoid getting hooked on a few favorites. You can become allergic to any food that you eat too frequently. Whether or not you are already food-allergic, a rotational diet is the safest and healthiest approach. The whole point of the diet is to allow the body to adjust to one food before consuming it again. If you eat wheat on Monday, for example, you should not eat it again for four days. It takes about that long for the body to recover from that exposure.

For a complete understanding of food allergies and how to avoid them, refer to Randolph and Moss's book *An Alternative Approach to Allergies*. (Also see Chapter 2 for a review of food allergies as related to panic and phobias.)

A Success Story

The Health Recovery System Clinic in Minneapolis, under the direction of Dr. Joan Mathews Larsen, provides its own special approach to nutrition and counseling and boasts an 85 percent recovery rate. The nutritional supplements used by that clinic are similar to those suggested here. It should always be emphasized that supplements are only part of an alcoholic's treatment program and should never be used exclusively.

My own experience with alcoholics who suffer from panic attacks and phobias has been that they are quickly able to control themselves once their fears are alleviated. This depends on a number of factors, of course. Those less severely addicted, especially females, seem to have the least difficulty with recovery. But, of course, unmotivated alcoholics cannot be treated successfully with any form of therapy.

Martha M., a patient of mine, first came to me because of her premenstrual syndrome. During the initial interview she revealed a chronic pattern of heavy alcohol consumption. Initially, she used alcohol to control the panic and intense anxiety prior to her period, but it gradually became a way of life. As her anxieties grew, so did her drinking. The alcohol she drank during her premenstrual phase so depleted her vitamin-mineral balance that she became more anxiety-prone during the rest of the month. The more alcohol she consumed to compensate for the new anxiety, the more her problem overlapped into her good days. Ultimately, there *were* no good days at all.

Martha's life seemed to be plagued by broken romances, short-lived jobs, and lost opportunities. At our first meeting she was just breaking up with another boyfriend and about to be terminated at work. She was hysterical, frightened, and emotionally unstable. By treating her for hypoglycemia as well as premenstrual syndrome with nutritional supplements, I was successful in reversing the process of panic and anxiety. Then I tested her for food allergies and removed certain foods from her diet to which she was allergy-addicted. At no time did I ever treat her for alcoholism. In time, she lost her desire to drink. When she did indulge on social occasions, emotional instability and depression returned. By this time, however, she recognized her symptoms as a food reaction and took steps to neutralize the problem. The last time I saw her, Martha had a steady job and a stable relationship, and most important, her drinking was under control.

7

How to Conquer the Panic and Fears Related to Anorexia, Bulimia, and Premenstrual Syndrome

You probably wonder why I have included this chapter in a book on fears and phobias. I have seen many patients with premenstrual syndrome who experience panic attacks while premenstrual and at no other time of the month. When their PMS is under control, so are the anxiety symptoms. Bulimics also suffer from a form of panic just after they have binged. The reaction that drives them to purge themselves or vomit the food they have just eaten is not exactly a classical form , but it definitely can be labeled as panic. Since patients with bulimia are often anorexic at times, I have included that disorder also. The fanatical way anorexics avoid food indicates a type of food phobia. This intense fear of food could also be described as a fear of ugliness, with obesity representing something unbearably repulsive. I will first discuss bulimia with a few additional thoughts about anorexia (some doctors consider them to be different phases of the same disease). Then I'll examine premenstrual syndrome.

ANOREXIA AND BULIMIA

Patients with both of these diseases have a significantly distorted body image. No matter what the scale says, or the mirror shows, the patient is absolutely convinced that he or she is oversized or obese. This pathological obsession with thinness exceeds all ranges of normality. Studies have shown that it is not unusual for people, especially young persons, to have distorted concepts of their appearance. This distortion often reflects their own estimates of self-worth. Studies show that such distortions of self-image tend to diminish with time and maturation and can also be "trained out" with structured therapy. In the case of true anorexics and bulimics, the distortions tend to resist change tenaciously. Any improvement that does occur is usually slow, and unless the efforts are continued, these individuals rapidly revert to their old obsessions.

Distorted self-concepts are one of the things eating-disorder patients have in common. There are a number of factors that separate them, however. The so-called primary anorexic has never been fat and is not inclined to binges. She will eat less even though she may feel hungry. There is a tendency on her part to deny herself pleasurable experiences (anhedonic). This type of anorexic is always thin or emaciated. As a group, they tend to be shy, retiring, and not very sexually active. They seldom come from families where obesity is prevalent.

A second group consists of people who usually have a family history of obesity. Unlike the primary anorexics, who were always thin, they were generally obese before the disease started. They are bulimic-anorexant, which means they have an abnormal interest in food at the same time as an abnormal interest in thinness. They equate the excessive desire to eat with being out of control.

This category of bulimic-anorexics also includes a fairly large number of individuals with other mental diseases. Many are involved with substance abuse: alcohol, amphetamines, and street drugs. Some are severely depressed. Most of them have higher than normal anxiety states, ranging all the way up to full-blown agoraphobia and panic. Many are compulsive, and it has been estimated that up to one third are kleptomaniacs.

In one study a third of the patients binged daily or more (Garfinkel 1981). As many as 80 percent ate vast quantities of food several times a week, sometimes repeatedly in one day. They felt intense guilt and panic and then induced vomiting. This group also seemed to be extremely impulsive, and, unlike the primary anorexics, were inclined to sexual promiscuity. Interestingly, there seemed to be a fairly high number who were kleptomaniacs. (Over 20 percent, in another report, were said to steal frequently.) They also reported frequent erratic mood swings.

Many bulimic patients, in spite of their excessive vomiting and excessive laxative use, never do become thin. Some have become alcoholics, some have attempted suicide, and others practice self-mutilation. Such persons, needless to say, have many characteristics of the addictive personality.

In one study (Hudson and Harrison 1983), about 50 percent of the patients had higher than normal cortisol levels, which is indicative of high stress. The authors of this same paper proposed that bulimia may be strongly connected to or may even signify a major mood disorder, particularly in cases of depression. These same authors closely studied the families of 75 bulimic patients and found the number of first-degree family members (mother, father, brother, sister) with similar mental problems was about the same as for a similar group of patients with major mood disorders. This leads to the conclusion that there may be a connection between bulimia and depression.

The Sugar Factor

Normal subjects do not enjoy the taste of sugar after they have eaten a large amount. Garfinkel found that obese bulimic patients do not experience this loss of interest in sugar the way a normal person does, nor did the anorexics who were tested. He also noted that the more anorexics overestimated and distorted their image of their own body size, the less they were deterred from eating more sugar after an initially large dose. The suggestion is clear, that anorexics are less responsive than normal people to internal cues that help the body maintain nutritional balance.

THE TREATMENT

The treatment for this illness is to restore both normal food intake and normal weight. Its purpose is also to put a stop to bingeing/purging and to restore some normality to self-image and self-appreciation. This has been accomplished by a number of methods, and psychopharmacological agents have been among the most significant.

Drugs to Treat Anorexia

Cyproheptadine (Periactin) is a serotonin antagonist and has long been known to stimulate weight gain. I have prescribed it for dozens of thin people who desired to put on pounds. It has also been used with success on patients with irritable bowel syndrome. The drug has also had some limited success with anorexics. At least a small percent of those who have used it have had increased appetites and weight gain. The dosage, up to 35 mg a day, can make some patients sleepy, since it is basically an antihistamine. It also has an antinauseant effect, and this may be one of its benefits. Some authors have theorized that a low-grade nausea sometimes contributes to anorexia. Because it is a prescription drug, your doctor will need to make the final decision. But it might be worth trying if panic is one of your symptoms. Antihistamines have assisted patients whose panic or fear symptoms may be related to inner-ear pathology (Levinson 1986).

A number of physicians have used up to 1,500 mg of lithium carbonate daily as a treatment for anorexia, especially if there was strong evidence of a severe mood disorder such as manic depression. Lithium has been beneficial to anorexics even without these strong signs of mood disorder (Gross and Ebert 1981), but researchers warn that unreliable, unstable, poorly managed patients could quickly develop a toxic condition if they continued restricted food intake, vomiting, and overusage of diuretics. So the benefits should be weighed against the risks.

Some time ago a strong tranquilizer, a dopamine blocker called chlorpromazine, was combined with bed rest and insulin injections and found to be moderately successful with anorexics. It was about 50 percent effective, and a second study using only chlorpromazine was also 50 percent successful. Since a side effect of many strong tranquilizers is weight gain, it is not surprising that anorexics do put on weight during treatment. Unfortunately, other side effects of these tranquilizers, most notably grogginess, cannot be tolerated by most patients.

Tricyclic antidepressants such as imipramine have enjoyed excellent success in cases of anorexia. The chronic deficiency of nutrients in anorexics has a significant effect on neurotransmitters, most notably on serotonin levels. These antidepressants will, in turn, have a countereffect, as a number of reports have confirmed. These reports reveal that both bulimic and anorexic patients are helped by the use of antidepressant MAO inhibitors such as phenelzine (Nardil). But in spite of their success, like lithium, they pose extreme dangers to poorly controlled patients.

Phenytoin (Dilantin) has also been used very successfully with bulimics and anorexics. Dilantin has been found to decrease binge-ing, and has helped bulimics more than anorexics. L-dopa supple-ments of one to three tablets daily have been tried with some success, but there has been no real research to support its efficiency.

The Nutritional Approach

ZINC

A journal article (*Lancet* 1984) reports the case of a thirteen-year-old girl with a diagnosis of anorexia nervosa who came to the clinic initially suffering from weight loss. She was given 15 mg of oral zinc daily, then this amount was increased to 50 mg three times a day. After four months, her weight increased by 30 lbs. and her depression improved considerably. When zinc was discontinued after ten months, the patient began to lose weight again and her depression returned. Zinc was given again, and within two months she was improving. Her reduced intake of food (the source of the original zinc deficiency) was probably due to a desire to keep her weight down in order to compete socially. But once zinc deficiency begins, it takes on a life of its own and devastates the patient's appetite and may precipitate depression.

Occasionally a dieting patient on a weight control program, who is not anorexic, will become fanatical about not eating and will deliberately drop below the recommended food allowance. Although concerned relatives usually encourage the patient to eat more, he or she generally doesn't respond and, in fact, becomes even more determined not to eat. It takes a great deal of effort to get these patients to resume a proper eating program. It should be noted that the type of patient most inclined to this phenomenon is the teenage female. There are reports of dieters not previously inclined to an-orexia who actually become triggered into it by weight control pro-grams.

I recently saw a fifteen-year-old girl who became suddenly an-orexic during such a program. She had lost all desire for food, but was not disturbed because she saw it as a perfect way to lose weight. Her parents, on the other hand, were much concerned and brought her in to see me. I found other symptoms of a zinc deficiency and I put her on 50 mg of zinc three times daily. Her desire for food returned within two days and continued as long as she took her mineral supplement.

The Brain Neurotransmitter System Is Very Important

The physiologies of appetite and satiety play a role in bulimia and these areas have also been targeted for treatment. The hypothalamus (discussed in Chapter 2) is the area of the brain where these centers are found.

The neurotransmitters involved in regulating these areas of the brain are already well known. The area of satiety in the hypothalamus contains multiple beta-adrenergic synapses that cause decreased hunger by inhibiting the feeding center. The neurotransmitter that activates this area is either adrenaline or noradrenaline. Another neurotransmitter, serotonin, also affects hunger; if serotonin goes down, hunger increases. An increase in L-dopa may also inhibit hunger, for these neurotransmitters are all balanced against each other. It's difficult to know what the exact balances should be, especially since they vary from one person to another. One research study has shown that imbalances of these neurotransmitters closely correlate to depression, and when the depression is improved, so is the neurotransmitter imbalance (Halmi 1985).

The amino acid (the neurotransmitter) that I have found most useful in this disease is GABA. I have used 500 mg three or four times daily with or without 7½ grams of ammonium chloride (a helper to GABA). Some patients have reported a remarkable drop in anxiety.

Other neurotransmitters that are useful are phenylalanine and tyrosine, which primarily block depression and serve as mild appetite suppressants. This helps the bulimic phase as it is helpful for bulimic patients to believe they have some control over their appetite. Control over cravings is also important, and my book *No More Cravings* (Warner Books, 1986) provides in-depth information on that subject.

I usually have my patients start with the first list of supplements below, then I add some items from the second list gradually if the initial supplements are not totally effective. If, after using both lists, control is not sufficient, I suggest they go back to Chapter 2 for more ideas on nutrition.

LIST 1

1. Zinc picolinate, 50 mg, 3 times daily
2. Niacinamide, 200 mg, 3 times daily and at bedtime; more may be used if necessary
3. B_6, 25 mg tablet 3 times daily
4. GABA, 500 mg tablet, 1 to 3 tablets 3 times daily; experiment with different levels
5. Ammonium chloride tablets, 7½ grams, 1 tablet 3 times a day
6. One good multivitamin-mineral supplement twice a day

LIST 2

1. Thiamine, 500 mg tablet 3 times a day
2. A complete amino acid capsule (containing all 22 amino acids) 3 times a day. (Try Aminoplex by Tyson.)
3. Choline, 1,000 mg 3 times daily
4. Calcium lactate, 500 mg 3 times daily
5. Tyrosine, 500 mg 3 times daily
6. Phenylalanine, 250 mg 3 times daily

Psychological Aspects

Anorexia nervosa has been described as a phobic aversion to food, or at least a perverse fear of obesity. It also appears to have obsessive-compulsive rituals as a component. Some believe that the phobias represent a symbolic method of maintaining self-control resulting from an internally originating sense of control loss. A parallel has been drawn between anorexia and the fear of contamination in that contaminants (in this case, foods) are considered to be harmful and are avoided at all costs. To anorexics, any caloric intake is considered detrimental in much the same way that germs are feared by obsessive compulsives. Obsessive-compulsive patients are realistic enough to know that what they are doing is irrational, but anorexics often do not see the irrationality of their fears. When patients are without any insight into their beliefs, it is difficult to find any point of contact for therapy.

Bulimia and anorexia nervosa were previously thought to be separate diseases, but now it is known that they frequently occur in the same subjects. It is easy to see this as a psychological problem since it exists mostly in the Western world where society is obsessed with thinness. It may or may not originate as a psychological problem, but it often ends up also being a physical one.

The psychological approaches to anorexia and bulimia have been reasonably good, especially when such treatment also includes support groups. But the physical approaches have also been of considerable benefit. As mentioned, zinc supplements have helped many, as have nutritional supplements given to reverse depression. Antidepressant drugs have also been useful, as well as drugs that stabilize sodium metabolism, such as Dilantin. A combined physical-psychological approach offers the greatest possibility of recovery to patients with these disorders.

PREMENSTRUAL SYNDROME

What Is PMS?

The average reader is probably aware of PMS. Numerous articles appearing in women's magazines and a flood of new books have discussed the subject in detail. But if you're still a little unsure, take this test:

BEFORE YOUR MENSTRUAL PERIOD DO YOU

	YES	NO
1. Seem to go crazy?	_____	_____
2. Get depressed?	_____	_____
3. Have difficulty smiling? Lose your sense of humor?	_____	_____
4. Become easily tired, fatigued?	_____	_____

	YES	NO
5. Experience increased hunger?	_____	_____
6. Crave sweets?	_____	_____
7. Feel mentally "off"?	_____	_____
8. Have strong mood swings?	_____	_____
9. Become irritable?	_____	_____
10. Become waterlogged, gain weight?	_____	_____
11. Notice breast soreness?	_____	_____
12. Get headaches?	_____	_____
13. Experience hypoglycemia (feel weak if you don't eat)?	_____	_____
14. Get acne, face breaks out?	_____	_____
15. Experience voice changes (hoarseness?)	_____	_____
16. Develop a bloated abdomen?	_____	_____
17. Notice that your joints become painful?	_____	_____
18. Get hay fever, runny nose?	_____	_____
19. Lose your sense of smell?	_____	_____
20. Experience dizziness?	_____	_____
21. Get bladder, urinary infections?	_____	_____
22. Get boils, sties, herpes?	_____	_____
23. Have increased desire for alcohol?	_____	_____
24. Notice that the same symptoms occur during ovulation (during the middle of your cycle)?	_____	_____
25. Have spasmodic symptoms, sometimes miss a period?	_____	_____

	YES	NO
26. Get colicky, have lower abdominal symptoms?	_____	_____
27. Experience painful intercourse at the time of your period?	_____	_____

Did you answer most of these questions yes? If so, you probably suffer from PMS. "But wait," you say. "A mere written test can't diagnose PMS. Aren't there laboratory tests that will give me a more concrete answer?" Actually, there aren't, but in the last three to five years, women's groups have aroused enough public interest to create pressure on the scientific community. The fervor is now strong enough to encourage more in-depth investigations into the problem.

PMS has always existed, but medical literature on the subject only goes back a scant fifty years. The symptoms of PMS, which seem endless, can begin as early as at ovulation (middle of the monthly cycle) and continue until the onset of menstruation, and sometimes beyond.

Beta-Endorphin

Giannini and his co-workers have proposed that women with PMS have less beta-endorphins than women who do not get PMS (Giannini and Price 1984). Normally, beta-endorphins increase during the premenstrual phase. Research has already determined that low levels of beta-endorphins are associated with depression and high levels are associated with manic states. It's easy to see how a rapidly fluctuating beta-endorphin level could be responsible for the psychological changes that occur during PMS.

The University of Illinois Medical Center has identified the major symptom of PMS to be a *local lack of self-control*. This control usually returns when menstruation begins. In my experience, however, I found that while symptoms often occur just before the menstrual period, they can actually show up any time of the month.

Psychological or Hormonal?

I have treated a large number of patients for PMS and one of the most common complaints I hear is "My family doctor says it's all in my head. He says there is no such thing as PMS." If a physician does take the patient seriously, he usually runs several general health tests and perhaps a few hormone tests and then, if they are normal, tells the patient, "I can't find anything wrong." As I mentioned, there are no reliable tests for PMS, so it is impossible for a doctor to make a definitive diagnosis, and thus the patient is still on her own, confused and frustrated.

Many clinicians believe that PMS is primarily a psychological disorder, but most research scientists disagree and lean toward hormonal dysfunction as the cause.

Men are often blind to what's happening. When a woman is irritable, depressed, or cross before her period, men often conclude that women use PMS as an excuse for bad behavior. Some men are so opinionated and close-minded that nothing can breach their impenetrable wall, and empathy and understanding don't exist.

Even women sometimes turn a deaf ear to their own problems. Full of doubt and guilt about PMS, they vacillate back and forth between accepting it as a physical occurrence and scolding themselves for being so weak. After all, shouldn't they be able to exert some self-control?

One thing appears consistent: The more "normal" a woman's biochemistry, the less PMS she will have, and the more abnormal her biochemistry, the greater her symptoms will be. I have found over 50 percent of the women with severe PMS also have symptoms of other biochemical imbalances, such as excessive fears and phobias, mucocutaneous candidiasis, strong allergic reactions to chemicals, and sometimes drug addictions.

Is There Anything That Triggers PMS?

1.   Tubal Ligation—A significantly large number of patients have complained to me that their PMS began directly after a tubal ligation. When I asked other doctors who treat PMS if they had received similar reports, their replies were positive. Although there are no in-depth studies to substantiate this, my own observations make it worthy of consideration.

2.   Birth Control Pills—Although the pill has been used to stop PMS, it is also possible that it may unbalance the hormones enough to be a causal factor. Many of my patients say their first symptoms began while they were on the pill.

3. Hysterectomy—A number of patients have reported symptoms similar to PMS after surgical menopause. These symptoms did not exist prior to the operation, but afterwards began occurring on a cyclic schedule once a month for one or two weeks. Fortunately, these cases usually respond extremely well to PMS treatment.

4. No Known Cause—One woman came to me complaining of PMS which she had experienced for the last nine months. It began without any apparent reason and had become progressively worse. I find that while more than half of my PMS patients can identify the trigger to their problem, a good number cannot.

Hunger and PMS

There are millions of women who crave foods only before their periods. The uncontrolled eating of chocolate, sugars, salt, and bakery products causes countless problems. Is it a physical occurrence, or is it imaginary? The study by Giannini and Price indicated a physical origin. Twenty patients kept a food diary for thirty days. Results indicated that not only did food intake increase during the PMS phase, but that it peaked along with other PMS symptoms. The authors suggested that it might be caused by an increase in the hormone called beta-endorphin.

Test for PMS

As stated, there are as yet no definitive tests that could conclusively state, "Mrs. Jones, you have PMS." However, there are tests that relate to the hormones that control the menstrual cycle. For example:

1. Prolactin—This hormone, related to the monthly cycle, has been found linked to PMS. If it's high, there are drugs you can take to lower it, but that isn't always the answer. I have seen a number of women whose high prolactin levels were lowered by the appropriate drug, and they still had PMS. Prolactin may be linked to PMS, but changing the levels doesn't necessarily halt cravings.

2.   Thyroid Hormones—The theory here is that a low thyroid level decreases proper ovulation and causes improper estrogen-progesterone ratios. This leads to PMS and cravings for chocolate and sweets. The treatment then would be to take thyroid medication, but my experience is that such treatment either doesn't help at all or it helps only minimally.

3.   FSH   (Follicle   Stimulating   Hormone),   LH   (Luteinizing Hormone)—These hormones are formed in the brain and are also responsible for estrogen-progesterone ratios. When they are not coordinated, the ratios become abnormal and PMS results. That's the theory, anyway. But whether they are unbalanced or not, their manipulation doesn't help the doctor control PMS or prevent premenstrual cravings.

4.   Estrogen and Progesterone Levels—An imbalance of these two hormones may be responsible for PMS. To correct this condition, progesterone may be given by injection and has been found to be very effective in relieving premenstrual cravings. I have never seen estrogen decrease PMS. In most cases, it only worsens the condition.

5.   Sex Hormone Binding Globulin (SHBG)—Katherine Dalton, M.D., has written an excellent book called *Once a Month* (Hunter House, 1979). In the book she describes the hormone SHBG. She believes a low level of this hormone may indicate a diagnosis of premenstrual syndrome, although not many experts agree with her.

Treatment for PMS

Psychologists have often attempted to connect premenstrual syndrome with various neuroses, preferring to believe that it occurs only in unstable women. Others state that mentally unstable individuals would naturally be more sensitive to any type of physiological change, either normal or abnormal (Gregory 1957). I have found some evidence of this in my patient population. The more neurotic the patient, the worse the symptoms and the more difficult to control. The more mentally stable the patient, the quicker the problem resolves itself, but PMS occurs in all ranges of mental states, normal or abnormal.

NUTRITIONAL TREATMENT OF PMS

Magnesium

One of the most commonly cited causes of PMS cravings is magnesium deficiency, yet blood tests on PMS patients seldom reveal it. Dr. Jeffery Blaud in his book *Nutraerobics* (Harper & Row, 1983) says that magnesium is low in the cells. When RBCs (red blood cells) are studied instead of the serum, the magnesium deficiency then becomes apparent.

Magnesium has also been helpful in relieving cramping that comes with menstruation. Two to four magnesium orotate tablets every time the cramping occurs has been reported effective. Those of us in preventive medicine have often used magnesium as a substitute for certain drugs. One of the drug groups that magnesium sometimes substitutes for are the calcium channel blockers.

One to three 100 mg magnesium tablets at the time a food craving occurs can be effective especially when reinforced by a 50 mg zinc tablet and a 50 mg B_6 tablet. One must be careful not to take amounts high enough to produce nervousness, for both B_6 and magnesium can cause hyperactivity.

Vitamin B_2

There is one other approach to PMS that I have used with some success. I prescribe 25 mg B_2 tablets and suggest that a patient chew one three times daily. This seems to work best when the PMS symptoms extend into the actual period. One important point: As soon as a patient regains control, I have her steadily reduce the number of tablets, until she can level off on the smallest amount that is effective, even if it's only half a tablet. Too much B_2, like any other vitamin, can unbalance the body's chemistry, thus causing further problems. Certain prescription drugs called calcium channel blockers are successful in the treatment of some PMS symptoms. In the cases reported, the greatest relief was found for symptoms of irritability, agitation, and emotional instability, including depression.

You'll have to see your family doctor for a prescription for this medication.

Essential Fatty Oils

Evening primrose oil has been called the "Queen of Vitamins." It contains essential fatty acids that help restore balance to the body. Take six to eight capsules daily for fourteen days before each period and one to three capsules at other times of the month. The effects are usually not felt initially, but after three to four months, you should notice a definite reduction in both PMS and cravings.

Evening primrose oil is frequently combined with vitamin E and other essential fatty acids to make up a good package. If you can find this combination, you should use twenty drops twice daily in liquid form, or take four to six capsules.

Vitamin B_6

This overtouted vitamin has helped a few poor souls, but not as much as its proponents would have you believe. Recently, I saw a patient who was instructed by her family physician to take 500 mg tablets of B_6 three times daily. I told her to discontinue it immediately, for B_6 in high doses can cause permanent neurological damage. Apparently the amount necessary for impairment is less than most experts have thought. A 1986 study reported nerve damage resulting from doses as low as 200 mg of B_6 daily for a year. I would not recommend B_6 in amounts greater than 50 mg three times a day, and then, only if one can see clear evidence of some benefit.

General Measures to Prevent PMS and Cravings

As you know, if you can prevent PMS, you can stop cravings. There are a number of good books that provide helpful suggestions. In addition, you can:

1. EDUCATE THE MAN IN YOUR LIFE

If he is not on your side, he may be working against you. There are plenty of inexpensive books on PMS for him to read. If he refuses to do so, go through a book yourself, underline the important parts, and read them to him. In other words, you must educate him even if it takes time. If he is already knowledgeable, ask him not to tempt you with sweets—especially when you are premenstrual. If he helps you resist these things, your battles will be more easily won.

2. DIET

Cutting down on carbohydrates during the premenstrual period greatly helps decrease PMS. That means no sugar or any sugary items. You should even eliminate fruits or restrict yourself to one serving daily—apples or cantaloupes are best. *No fruit juices.* A common mistake is to think that concentrated fruit juices are healthy. They do contain nutrients, but they also flood sugar into the body, and, like refined sugar, they cause more water retention than salt.

3. CAFFEINE, COFFEE, TEA, COLAS, CHOCOLATE

All of these rob the body of water-soluble vitamins through diuresis or by being metabolized out. In addition, these items may cause hypoglycemia. There is absolutely no doubt that caffeine intensifies PMS.

4. ALCOHOL

Alcohol is essentially pure sugar and behaves like sugar in the body. It causes the same problems as sugar, and often more intensely.

5. FOOD ALLERGIES

Use Chapter 4 to uncover any food allergies, then do not eat those foods during your premenstrual time. Each of these foods may disturb your hormone balance just as severely as sugar or caffeine.

6. EXERCISE

A number of patients have reported relief of premenstrual symptoms by embarking on a heavy exercise program during the last two weeks of each cycle. That means three to five one-hour sessions each week. Even if you don't get total relief, you will benefit in a number of important ways from a regular exercise program.

8

How to Conquer the Fears of Flying, Heights, and Driving

Some of the people who sit at airport bars swigging double martinis don't normally drink. They are using alcohol in a last-ditch effort to calm themselves enough to get on the plane. Once in flight, they may have a few more stiff ones to fortify themselves until they're back on the ground again. It has been estimated that 25,000 Americans perceive airplanes as little more than flying coffins.

Sometimes such fears originate after an unpleasant flying experience. Bad weather can be hair-raising, especially if the wind tosses the plane around like a piece of plywood. During one such rough encounter when the plane was bouncing violently, a passenger next to me was talking to a pilot hitching his way home. She asked him what was keeping the plane up, and how it could survive heavy turbulence. He patiently explained every detail to her in the simplest terms, from takeoff to landing, including the nature of air currents and the design and stability of planes built to withstand all these elements. I thought he did a thorough and convincing job. After he was through, I turned to my seatmate and said, "Well, what do you think now?" She answered, "Oh, he explained it all to me quite clearly. But I didn't believe a word he said."

A Question of Control

This woman's concern, like most people's, was that once one is strapped into an airplane seat, it is no longer possible to control one's destiny. Every new sound of the engine, every tilt of the plane, every variation of speed, causes a rush of panic. Unfortunately, there is usually no one around to explain these normal changes and no one to tell the panicked person how to cope. Rough weather and a rough landing only make matters worse. If a first flight is an "eventful" one, it doesn't make the next one any easier. At the end of one of my flights we were landing in Cozumel, Mexico. A thundering rainstorm reduced visibility to almost zero just as we were about to touch down. It was clear, however, that we were hundreds of yards short of the runway and would face a water landing. The pilot punched his engines, and the plane somehow stayed up long enough to make the runway. Near accidents like this are not uncommon. The reality is that there *are* risks to flying.

In the many years that I have been a passenger, I have had a number of such experiences, and yet I continue to fly. Not because I thrive on the thrill of near accidents, but because I know that pilots are intelligent individuals, well trained, and as eager to live as I am. When there is a potential problem, they quickly make necessary adjustments, and everything usually turns out fine. Although errors frequently occur, built-in safety factors cover 99 percent of all these possibilities. It's because of these incredible safety backups that flying is virtually as safe as staying home, and statistically safer than driving to the store.

It's not so much the fear of dying that frightens most people, but rather the fear of being out of control. A feeling of total helplessness accompanies exposure to danger when there are literally no options in case of trouble. In a car or train, you might manage to jump out, and in a bus you might get under a seat. In an airplane there's absolutely nothing you can do except follow the pilot's instructions.

How I Overcame My Fear of Flying

I overcame my fear of flying without using any of the devices that I'm going to recommend to you. I used to sit at the window of an airplane and look straight down. Then I'd begin to fantasize some grim catastrophe. I'd imagine the door of the plane flying open and my being sucked out into the whirling clouds. How horrible to fall screaming for eternity to certain death below! After I exhausted this daydream, I would imagine other flaws in the plane. Perhaps all the bolts on the wing were faulty. Some years ago, I actually saw a wing fall off of an airplane in flight. It could happen again. I could just see a cabinful of people screaming hysterically as the plane plummeted crazily toward earth and finally crashed in a burst of flames.

I would go on like this for hours, contriving all sorts of horrible ways to die. If there was a sudden strange noise, like the flaps changing position, of course I'd imagine the worst. And if the plane wobbled a little as we were landing, I'd brace myself for disaster. My every thought caused me to sweat, and my heart would race wildly. In some futile way I was trying by mind and body to do the impossible—to control the flight. Of course each trip was sheer terror. Finally, exhausted by all this self-inflicted torture, I decided to try something new. I decided that I would start controlling my emotions properly, not haphazardly, as each feeling developed.

First of all, I realized that I was experiencing anxiety, tenseness, and nervousness. Nature's purpose in creating those feelings is to stimulate the endangered animal to act, to serve as a sort of cattle prod that won't stop poking until action is taken. If I didn't do something, the feelings would remain and make me uncomfortable, even prevent me from functioning normally. Beginning at the simplest level, I began to ask myself questions: Did I have anxiety because of the flight? Yes! It wasn't there before the flight and nothing else had occurred in the meantime. What was I worried about? I didn't want to die, and I was worried that I might. There are risks in air travel and, although small, they *are* very real. What were my options? I could refuse to fly and avoid my fears, but that would result in a great deal of inconvenience. My life-style would be restricted and I wouldn't be able to do half the things I wanted. Finally, I realized the *real* problem wasn't flying. The real problem was me. I had trouble with anxiety every time I left the ground.

I knew that flying was safer than driving a car. So what was my problem? What was my real, bottom-line problem? The answer was that I was afraid to put my life totally, unconditionally, into the hands of another person. I didn't trust those who built the planes. I had no confidence in the mechanics who checked it over, and though I knew that pilots are well screened, highly trained, and experienced, I guess I had reservations about them too. The fact is that airplanes are tested and retested until it's virtually impossible for them to be defective. At regular intervals, necessary or not, government regulations call for still more inspections. How many more safety precautions can you ask for? All these fail-safe procedures make mechanical failures extremely rare. Most accidents are due to weather or chance, and their incidence is dramatically low compared to the number of flights and hours in the air.

I had to admit that it came down to me—I couldn't improve on the pilots or the planes, so I needed to start seeing and thinking differently. Suppose I actually was going to crash, die, let's say two hours after takeoff. If I had only a couple of hours left, did I want those last two precious hours filled with terror and futile attempts to control the uncontrollable? Or did I want my last moments to be filled with fun, laughter, interesting stories, and perhaps a good cigar? Let death come suddenly, without warning. If I only had two hours left, I wanted to be feeling good right to the end.

So I set out to change my thought patterns. Every time I began on one of my catastrophe fantasies, I would deliberately focus my attention on a magazine article. If I felt myself becoming nervous, I tried to concentrate on what others around me were doing. *I simply relinquished all desire to want to change and control things.* Realistically, I could change nothing anyway, so it served no purpose to worry about lack of control. Therefore, I made a bargain with myself to block out all worry. Every time the panic started, I would intervene, saying to myself, "Well, here you go again. Is there anything about this situation you have control over?" Answer: No. There is no point in worrying about something you can't control. So I would continue to find ways to distract myself, and the more often I successfully diverted my attention, the fewer times I broke out in a cold sweat. Soon I began to enjoy flying and using my time productively.

I know this is a very hard concept for people who insist on always being in control of their lives, but flying is simply one of those areas where control is impossible. It's sometimes good for a highly controlling person temporarily to give up his power, to surrender completely, to submit passively to reality.

A Good Attitude Is Essential

First of all, it helps to know that everyone, including the flight crew, experiences some degree of nervousness at takeoff. Even though the man across from you seems intent on reading the paper, he is probably as relieved as you when the plane is safely in the air. The stewards can easily hide any concern they might have by seeing to the passengers' comfort. The pilot, although sure of himself, may still alleviate a little normal anxiety by double-checking his instruments. A certain amount of nervousness on the part of everyone on board is both normal and expected. Excessive fear, on the other hand, is neurotic.

It has been said that people who frighten easily have especially vivid imaginations. They create "disaster films" in their heads, often forgetting that possibilities are not probabilities. Every time a plane takes off, it is *possible* that something could go wrong, but the probabilities are far removed. Statistically it's highly unlikely that you will actually take that well-rehearsed plunge to disaster.

Too many people try to use their emotions as "magic" to control the plane and the crew. As one lady said, "In my mind I was trying to stop the plane from taking off." She learned, as we all eventually do, that we can't control the plane. The only things we can control are our own emotions and thoughts. Once we let go of our need for external control and begin to work on our emotions, our fears start to disappear.

A secondary problem connected with air travel is feeling trapped in a cabin full of people. Those inclined to claustrophobia, or fear of enclosed places, have an additional reason to become nervous. Such individuals must use whatever coping techniques they've mastered to deal with those fears before they can even consider combating the fear of flying.

Fortunately, the formula for the fear of flying usually takes care of both problems. Take the formula below, one hour before taking off.

The Nutritional Treatment

1. Start with
   Calcium lactate, 500 mg
   Tryptophan, 1,000 to 1,500 mg
   You may add:
   B_1, 500 mg
   Choline, 2,000 mg
   Biotin, 5000 mcg
   Aspirin, 5 grains

2. "Extra Strength" formula:
   Calcium lactate, 2,000 mg
   B_1, 500 mg
   Choline, 2,000 mg
   Biotin, 5000 mcg
   Aspirin, 300 mg
   Pantothenic acid, 1,000 mg

3. Doses may be repeated every four hours during flight.

4. For twenty-four hours prior to leaving, avoid the following: Caffeine, sugar (including fruits), alcohol, and recreational drugs. If you use any of these substances, it will totally undermine the formula. You should also get a full night's sleep before flying with the help of one or two tryptophan tablets and the use of relaxation exercises.

If your problem is a simple fear of flying, all that's needed is a little help, but if the problem is compounded by a number of other fears, ranging all the way up to full-blown agoraphobia, then treatment should not be attempted until you are also successfully dealing with these other anxieties. If you are a practicing alcoholic, it's unlikely that this treatment will be of any benefit until you achieve sobriety.

You may get rewarding results with the nutritional formula, but if you want complete independence, then you will need to face your fears over and over again until they are finally conquered. If your fears are overwhelming, then try the easy way first—do it all in your imagination. To make it easier on yourself, take the nutritional formula an hour before doing the following exercise.

Desensitization Technique

Go into a quiet, dimly lighted room and sink into a soft easy chair. Use the relaxation techniques described in Chapter 4, then go through a series of scenes using imagery. Close your eyes, then as vividly as possible imagine scenes that cause you anxiety. If any particular fear persists, keep repeating the scene until you can experience it without discomfort. When you can easily handle the scene, go into the next one. Each practice session should last about fifteen to twenty minutes. You may practice once every day or several times a day, but always start with scene one and continue through the other scenes as rapidly as possible, stopping when you begin to feel nervous. Keep working that scene until you feel anxiety-free. When you are totally comfortable, progress to the next scene until each one can be repeated in sequence, without distress.

1. Begin by thinking about taking a flight. Don't imagine the plane ride itself, just the idea that you might fly somewhere.

2. Now you've definitely decided to take the trip. You go to the phone, call the travel agency, and order the tickets. You've set the time, date, and details, and things are under way. If necessary, pick a specific destination, such as a dream vacation you've always fantasized about.

3. It's now the day of the trip. Pack your bags. Decide in detail what you are going to take: shoes, clothes, coats, underwear, toiletries, cosmetics, magazines, presents for anyone you're visiting. Also, plan for your transportation to and from each airport.

4. Call for a taxi or get your car ready to go, turn out the lights, set the alarm, or whatever other final preparations are necessary. Now slowly start your drive. See the streets one by one as you leave your neighborhood. Now turn into a major street; now get onto the freeway.

5. You are finally approaching the airport. It's a mile away, but you can see the signs directing you to the parking or unloading area. Now you park, and unload your bags. You enter the lobby and go to the ticket counter. After a wait in line, you get your tickets and check your luggage.

6. Walk through the security gate and down the hall toward the waiting area. Get your seat assignment and sit down with the rest of the passengers.

7. You hear the announcement "Passengers may board now," as the line forms to enter the plane. Your ticket is taken, and you walk down the ramp to the doorway of the plane. The flight attendants smile as you enter, and you find your way to your seat. You place your hand luggage overhead, then sit down and buckle your seat belt.

8. Everyone is on board. The doors are closed and the safety announcements are given over the speaker, as the plane slowly taxis to takeoff. Everyone around you seems to be calm, talking and smiling. They all appear as relaxed and unconcerned as you are. The plane is now on the runway, waiting for permission to take off.

9. Slowly the plane taxis down the runway, gradually picking up speed. You look around. The other passengers are reading or talking, just as relaxed as you are. As the plane lifts off the ground, you hear several loud noises as the wheels are brought up under the plane. It's noisy, but a normal sound during takeoff.

10. Once off the ground, the usual cabin activity takes place; cocktails are served, seat belts are unbuckled, No Smoking signs flicker off, and some people go to the bathroom, while others begin to read or talk.

11. At first the flight is calm and uneventful. But suddenly, the plane encounters turbulence. It begins to bounce and vibrate. High-altitude air currents are uneven, and as the plane flies through them, it continues to lurch. All airplanes are built to easily withstand this kind of normal turbulence. You don't need to concern yourself. It's all to be expected, and the plane is in no danger. This rough spell should last only a few minutes, then you'll be in smooth air again.

What to Expect from Treatment

- If fear of flying is your only major fear, then it can be controlled with relative ease.
- If you are agoraphobic or have a number of compounding fears, then it will take more time and patience to achieve results.
- Agoraphobia and multiple phobias should be treated at the same time as fear of flying, or a good outcome will not be likely.

FEAR OF HEIGHTS

Some people are so afraid of heights that even if they are only three feet off the ground, they develop an overwhelming feeling of being drawn toward the edge, and in some cases feel a compulsion to jump. Some experts believe this is a release of an inner need for self-destruction. Others feel it's a need to put an end to fear by taking drastic action. Some older theories have even suggested a need to fly, without regard for consequences. A number of psychiatrists think fear of heights is symbolic of all basic insecurities, while still others consider it to be a fear of a loss of symbolic superiority or the feeling that one does not "deserve" to be elevated.

Children who crawl already have a fear of falling and tend to avoid edges or raised areas. Older people and invalids can be in the same category, for they often risk injury by slipping off balance. Often the causes of this phobia can be traced to a serious fall or near fall. Unlike those with normal survival instincts, phobics don't just worry about falling, they *know* they will. Those able to work on high-rise projects obviously have the opposite feeling; they are confident they will *not* fall. It's a matter of attitude and belief.

Treating Fear of Heights

EXERCISE 1—ROLE PLAYING

It should be kept in mind that changing one's behavior can change one's life faster than merely altering one's thoughts. Clients are often surprised to hear a therapist say, "If you don't feel happy, then pretend you're happy, act as if you are." The patient may think his therapist is suggesting that he be phony or insincere, but in reality, the premise is that by behaving a certain way, your thoughts and feelings will eventually coincide with your actions, and in time will catch up with them until you actually *are* happy.

The same is true of courage or peace of mind. Action can be the starting point of change. Move and act the way you would like to be, and sooner or later your thoughts and emotions will fall into line. Many a young actor who sees himself in the makeup of an old man has been surprised to find himself beginning to think and feel like a senior citizen. He soon finds that he is pretending less and less as he gets deeper into his role. In therapy, the same principles apply. When you are in a fearful situation, try pretending you are not afraid. If you pretend hard enough, you will find that, almost magically, your fears will begin to fade. At this point, review Chapter

4 and give particular attention to the section on Paradoxical Intention. Use that technique combined with role playing, and you will find that you get almost immediate relief from your fears.

EXERCISE 2—GRADUAL EXPOSURE

1. Select an apartment or commercial building twelve to twenty-five stories high. It must have a fire escape or other balconies which are accessible from the inside. You may go from floor to floor by either elevator or stairs.

2. Start out on the first floor. Walk to the rail and stop for ten to twenty seconds, then go back in and up one flight more.

3. A friend should stand at the bottom to give you advice and support.

Remember these important points:

- Follow this sequence as rapidly as possible.
- Go through the steps regardless of how upset you feel or what thoughts you have while doing the exercise.
- Ignore your thoughts and feelings as much as possible. Just go through the motions.
- Continue for an hour or until you have reached the top of the building.
- If you were not able to reach the top, then start your next hour session at the last floor that you were successful in reaching.
- If you feel you must come down, your friend should be supportive but firm, and send you back up to try again.
- Take supplements listed under "Fear of Flying" 60 to 90 minutes before each session.
- After you have reached the top, the treatment is over. Most people can usually do this within a session or two.

EXERCISE 3—BREATH HOLDING

A case report tells of a patient whose fear of stairs was removed in one therapy session (Etkin 1973). With her back to a stairwell, the woman was asked to close her eyes and exhale all the air from her lungs. Then, she was told to hold her breath as long as she could. When she had almost reached the point where she could no longer hold it, she signaled the therapist, who turned her around so she faced the stairs, still with her eyes closed and her breath held. She was instructed to continue not breathing, which was only possible for a few seconds more. Her eyes were then opened and she was allowed to take in air. The flood of relief at being able to breathe again totally overwhelmed the fear of the stairs. The procedure was repeated, and soon the patient felt free of her phobia.

This type of exercise would, of course, require an assistant. Another method would be to stand at the base of a stairway with your back toward it. Hold your breath until it is impossible to hold it any longer, then, while breathing, turn around and climb a few stairs. This could be repeatedly done over a period of thirty minutes to an hour. Combined with nutritional supplements, it is possible to "train out" some phobics within an hour. The assistant must be careful, however, to make sure that the patient doesn't become faint during the breathing exercise.

FEAR OF DRIVING

Fear of driving is an isolated phobia, a single and immediate fear, while fear of flying or heights seems often to be a symptom of higher than normal fear levels, or other basic insecurities.

Fear serves many purposes, but its primary function is to keep us alive. Since life itself depends on the food chain, each group of organisms represents one link. Human beings, like most other animals, are both predator and prey. Fear is a necessary instinct that enables us to avoid our predators (which now, for our species, is usually our fellow man). We are now discussing, of course, genuine reasons to be afraid. In instances of sudden danger, most organisms react with blind preprogrammed survival reflexes. Our hand pulls away from a hot stove before our mind has a chance to sort through the alternatives.

Supposedly, these reflexes are set up to deal with and protect us from imminent destruction. Modern life, however, isn't that simple. These reflexes "go off" even when we merely suspect that we *might* be in danger. They may spontaneously discharge in an animal who detects a twig breaking nearby which could signal a stalking predator ready to pounce, or a shadow falling on the edge of his range of vision. Often, triggers go off in the presence of something unexpected. The "shock" not only surprises us, but it may also "condition" us and leave a permanent memory in our nervous system, so that we are better prepared the next time.

Pavlov

Pavlov was the first to show how easy it is to train animals to avoid things. He trained their nervous systems to associate pain or fear of pain with a particular object. In this way, the animal could be made to avoid the object, or conversely, if positive conditioning had been conducted, the animal would learn to seek out the object. Theoretically, if an animal makes a mistake and overreacts to a nonthreatening object or situation, it could then reason out or see the mistake and correct its behavior. Ideally, it should become more realistic about what is really dangerous and what has proved to be an unfounded fear. If everything went according to the book, that's what would happen; but what we see occurring, in both men and animals, is the permanent programming within the nervous system of these "mistakes."

It has been found that well-trained fear responses linger on even after hundreds of repeated experiences in which there is no threat from the original object or location.

How does this happen? First of all, we know that such responses do occur because the original fearful situation can be repeatedly evoked in patients with single phobias, for instance, a young girl still afraid of horses after being nearly killed by one at the age of six. It may on the other hand take several such episodes before overresponsiveness occurs, but eventually such conditioning takes place. Not in everyone, but in certain predisposed individuals.

Many Ways to Become Afraid

There are many ways a person can become afraid of an object or situation. It can happen through a fearful experience, or by observing others' fears, or by simply being told that something is dangerous.

Fear of lightning, for example, usually originates from personal experience, while the fear of earthquakes frequently comes not only from personal experience, but from observing panic in others. Fear of snakes can develop from printed information or from stories about unfortunate victims. In one study, 30 patients were asked how they developed their phobias about driving (Munjack 1984). At the time of the interview, none of the subjects were able to drive freeways, and twenty-two had some trouble even driving local streets. Twelve had panic attacks while on the freeways, and six had freeway collisions. Three others reported unusually frightening experiences while on the road. Four others developed fears after severe family stresses. Two patients had a long history of driving phobias and out of the thirty, only one could not explain how his fears originated.

My Fear of Driving

Some years ago, I was driving the freeway when a line of cars in front of me suddenly stopped. I hit my brakes but was hurled toward the car in front of me. An accident seemed inevitable, but somehow, I managed to find a clear space in an adjacent lane and swerved into it just in time to avoid a disastrous collision. I was so frightened that I got off the freeway and slowly drove home on local streets. The next day as I entered the freeway, I found myself a nervous wreck. Instead of pulling into the fast lane as was my habit, I stayed in the slow lane and drove like a little old lady. If I got within a quarter mile of the car in front, I became terrified that I would not be able to control my car. Rationally, I knew this was ridiculous because I had plenty of time in which to stop; yet my fear was overwhelming, and it intensified every time I got too close to another car.

From professional experience, I knew I had to keep driving and work my way through these fears, but I still continued to exercise undue caution—to the considerable irritation of the drivers around me. It took almost two years for my anxiety to be completely resolved. Unfortunately, this incident occurred before I was aware of the nutritional factors that could have saved me a great deal of grief.

Usually, there is a traumatic occurrence that causes anxiety to arise on cue. It has been suggested (Munjack 1984) that the necessity of being in control of a car contributes to the intensity of the attack.

Trauma occurs when control is threatened. Afterwards, there continues to be not only a high level of fear, but a real need to avoid any position of possible entrapment.

Two years later, I experienced an even closer call. Once again a car in front of me stopped suddenly to avoid a disabled car. When I hit my brakes, they failed completely. I grabbed my emergency brake, but it was too late. I swerved away from a collision, but lost control of my car as it skidded across all five lanes of the freeway. By some stroke of luck, drivers in the other lanes were alert enough to avoid me, but it could easily have become a demolition derby with tragic results. I found myself completely turned around facing oncoming traffic in the fast lane. Miraculously, the cars slowed and stopped for me, and I whirled my car around and resumed my journey, trying to function normally and act nonchalant. I kept whistling and adjusting my radio as cars passed by, their drivers staring. What was the result of this near catastrophe? Nothing! Surprisingly enough, I did not develop a phobia.

I'm not sure why on one occasion I became phobic and in another, even more intense incident, I did not. What I suspect is that we all have windows of vulnerability, created by hormonal and biochemical balances so that we are more easily imprinted at one time than another.

NUTRITIONAL TREATMENT FOR THE FEAR OF DRIVING

One hour prior to driving a car, take these items:

1. B_1, 500 mg
2. Choline, 1,000 mg
3. Calcium lactate, 500 mg
4. Niacinamide B_6, 2,000 mg
5. Mintran, 3 tablets (see page 175)

If this formula does not completely suppress your fears, then add some of the ingredients from the "fear of flying" formula. If you've been driving but avoiding the freeways or driving in an overly cautious fashion, then the formula should help bolster your courage. If, on the other hand, you have been avoiding driving altogether, then it might be easier to ease back into it with the exercise below.

Set up the following series of driving tasks:

SUGGESTED TASKS

1. Drive twelve blocks down a quiet residential street.
2. Drive twelve blocks down a slightly busy street.
3. Drive twelve blocks through a commercial district.
4. Drive three miles on a highway (not a freeway).
5. Drive three miles on a freeway at a time when traffic is light.
6. Drive eight miles on a crowded freeway.

RULES

- You must do the thing that you wish to avoid.
- You must do it no matter how badly you feel or how many negative thoughts you've had. Concentrate on ignoring these feelings and focus your energies on the job at hand.
- Have a friend follow you in another car.
- Take your vitamins 60 to 90 minutes before driving.
- Practice sessions should last an hour. When one task is completed, go on to the next and continue until all the tasks are completed.
- At the end of an hour, if all tasks are not completed, stop anyway. Start the next session with the last task you finished successfully, then continue for the rest of the hour.
- The treatment is over after you can do all six tasks, but you may continue to practice if you find it helpful.

9

How to Conquer Social Phobias

There are certain types of anxieties that are similar to phobias, and yet they cannot be clinically classified as such. These fears are found in so many people, it's hard to know when a patient has crossed the line into the area of a disease. Shyness is a common example, and many persons who have been described as "painfully shy" often do not seek professional advice. This is unfortunate, because extremely shy people do need help; and if they don't get it, they often lead lonely lives and miss out on important opportunities.

Social phobia, a fear of people, ranges from nonassertive behavior to being a "loner," and all the way to classic paranoia. Needless to say, such a fear can stunt one's growth in all areas of life and, like shyness, is embarrassing to talk about.

Fear of looking ugly is another area I have included because it's so common. It's rare that people feel that they look as good as they would like. Almost all of us are concerned with how we appear to others, realizing that, to some extent, social value depends on physical attractiveness. All you have to do is look at the sales figures of cosmetics companies to understand how important it is for people to feel they look their best. But, like all attitudes and self-concepts, this anxiety can be carried to extremes.

Worry is another universal phenomenon. We fear not having enough money, losing our job, our looks, our friends, and so on. Each of these fears is not something we necessarily share with others; sometimes we keep them to ourselves, and, sadly, we pay a price for being overly sensitive.

It's especially difficult to talk about things like rape or assault— victims often find it painful to fully acknowledge such traumas— but if we don't deal with these fears, we drag them along with us, and they become a cross to bear for the rest of our lives. Fortunately, rape centers and victim support groups are growing in number and offer help dealing with the emotional consequences of crime.

SOCIAL PHOBIAS

Fear that makes a person avoid social situations is quite common in adolescence, but is usually overcome in the course of growing up. As we gain maturity, shyness recedes, and social situations become more enjoyable. For some persons, however, social fear persists and can range from avoiding specific social occasions to the shunning of all new relationships. This may be the source of the so-called "loner syndrome" with all its attendant problems. Often it involves a fear of authority figures, older people, and employers, and it may extend to a fear of crowded rooms or even the entire opposite sex.

Unreasonable Anxieties

Social phobias also include an irrational fear of scrutiny by others, a fear of embarrassment or humiliation, which can range from anxieties about talking on the telephone to public speaking. In severe cases, a person may become a virtual hermit. This unreasonable anxiety experienced in the company of others often increases with the formality of a given situation, as well as the degree of scrutiny or observation.

There is a normal social anxiety that all of us experience. Who isn't just a bit shy on occasion; who doesn't have trouble saying no to unreasonable requests? Who among us is not anxious, if only a little, when he must speak to an audience? Some degree of social phobia exists in all of us, but it usually doesn't take over our lives. True social phobics can be so disabled by their fears that they become housebound. If their jobs force them out on a daily basis, then they become prisoners on weekends. One such patient said, "I always imagined people were critical of me. I worried what they thought about me. These fears filled me with a lack of self-confidence.

My head was always down, and my shoulders were slumped. I could never look anyone straight in the eye. If I saw someone I knew coming along the street, I would cross to the other side so I wouldn't have to speak as I passed. A roomful of people would throw me into a panic, and I would leave quickly. I even hesitated answering the phone. You'll never know how lonely and depressed I felt."

Because of their avoidance behavior, most severe social phobics are unable to relate well to others. They lack social skills; their gestures are clumsy, and they are totally unable to express their feelings. Such behavior forces them inward so that they rely a lot on daydreams and worry about being "wallflowers." Social phobias usually develop from puberty to the age of thirty, more frequently in males than females.

Overwhelming fears in social situations often lead to more specific fears such as fear of blushing, fear of vomiting, fear of trembling, fear of fainting, and fear of authorities. The fear of eating and drinking in public is disturbing but not generally as severe as the dread of vomiting. Such patients are constantly *searching the environment for anyone around who looks as though he might* get sick. At the same time, they check around to be sure they will be able to escape if necessary.

Agoraphobia is sometimes confused with severe social phobia, but there are enough differences so that accurate diagnoses can readily be made.

AGORAPHOBIA	SOCIAL PHOBIA
Symptoms begin in the late teens or twenties	Symptoms begin in preteens or early teens
The majority of reported cases are female	The majority of reported cases are male
No special social class	Usually from higher social class
Definitely related to family history and genetics	Phobia not commonly found in these families
Excessive use of alcohol reported	Excessive use of alcohol reported
Starts after a trauma or sudden panic attack	Starts gradually, often goes unnoticed for a time
Often mixed with other phobias	Seldom phobic in other ways

If you have many of the symptoms I have been discussing, and you wonder if you have a social phobia, then take the following test:

                                    YES   NO

1. I don't like being teased.   _____   _____

2. I dislike public transportation.   _____   _____

3. I get scared when I meet people
   with authority.   _____   _____

4. I don't like to cross streets.   _____   _____

5. I hate being watched when I'm
   doing something.   _____   _____

6. I don't like to be alone.   _____   _____

7. I don't enjoy using the telephone. _____   _____

8. I dislike going to department
   stores.   _____   _____

9. I do not want others to watch when
   I am writing something.   _____   _____

10. I don't like unfamiliar places.   _____   _____

11. I don't like to entertain visitors. _____   _____

12. I don't like crowds.   _____   _____

13. I don't like to eat at home with
    other people.   _____   _____

14. I don't like small, enclosed shops. _____   _____

15. I hate to speak in public.   _____   _____

16. I can't stand open places.   _____   _____

17. I blush often.   _____   _____

18. My limbs get weak when I get ner-
    vous.   _____   _____

19. My muscles twitch when I'm ner-
    vous.   _____   _____

20. When I'm nervous my ears ring or
    buzz.   _____   _____

If many of your yes answers were to odd-numbered statements, you have a tendency to be a social phobic. If you answered over seven of the odd-numbered statements yes, you probably do suffer from social phobia. If you answered most of the even-numbered statements yes, you lean toward agoraphobia. Although these groups at times share common symptoms, there is a clear distinction between the two disorders. Agoraphobics are less sensitive and not so afraid with others; in fact, they often feel better in the presence of other people. What they avoid is crowded open areas away from home. Social phobics, on the other hand, are mainly afraid of people-contact, be it at home or in public places. They are particularly bothered when they are being observed by others.

Shyness

There are many terribly lonely people in close proximity to others who would cherish some company. The trouble is, they can't force themselves to make the first contact.

How do people get this way? Some doctors believe that people may be born with this tendency, because they seem to come from families that have a high susceptibility to threatening situations. These people are wiped out by even the most inconsequential rejections. Their inborn tendency to overreact in social situations can be made better or worse by environmental factors. In some, shyness just seems to burn itself out with time. Others, however, because of a passive nature, continue to reinforce the inappropriate behavior and never develop poise or social ease.

Another aspect to shyness is selfishness. Through withdrawal, we can escape from the pains of life, and we can hide from our own unpleasant feelings by indulging in fantasy. If we do not get involved with others, we can do what we want without being obligated or responsible. Shyness has a positive appeal to some people who don't want to be lonely and forgotten, but often don't want to give up their selfish ways either.

General Approaches to Social Phobias

Here are several methods that have been successfully used to treat these phobias. Look them over and choose the one best for you.

1. Keep a day-to-day diary of your progress. In the journal, write down your goals and when you think you will deal with them. Start with interpersonal relationships. Make a list from the least fearful to the worst possible situation. Make your first goal the easiest and proceed to the most difficult. For example:

- Ask a stranger for change
- Ask someone for a date

Variation: Some therapists suggest using a bit of pressure. List several things you enjoy doing such as watching TV, then do not allow yourself any television, until you have reached your goal for the day.

2. Seek out a support group. Social phobics do better when they have group support and a place to practice in relative safety.

3. Set some personal improvement goals:

- More eye contact
- Better conversational ability
- Improved body posture and more "open" body language

4. Try standing back from your problem and taking a long objective look. Will any of the things you are worried about matter to anyone in fifty years? Do people really care as much as you think?

Methods of Handling Anxiety

1. RELAXING

a. Learn how to relax; use the techniques described in Chapter 4.
b. After you have practiced enough to be able to relax completely, associate a cue word with this sensation. Pick a word that appeals to you such as *warm, calm, relaxed,* etc. Begin your relaxation procedure, and when you sense you are completely tranquil, use your cue word for twenty consecutive exhalations. Rest a minute or two and then do it again. Try to increase your level of relaxation with each cue word.
c. Rehearse relaxation and cue words daily for thirty days.
d. After four weeks of practice, try the cue word in a situation

when you are mildly anxious. If successful, continue to practice under different sets of circumstances.

2. STOPPING YOUR THOUGHTS

You may use this technique directly in real-life situations, or you may wish to practice first. I assure you it will work. I've used this technique successfully on many patients. Its purpose is to help you stay in the solution, not in the problem.

- a. Find an easy chair in a quiet room.
- b. Close your eyes and relax.
- c. Start to think about your fears, getting right to the point. Don't intellectualize. Don't be analytical; rather, be as dramatic and close to your feelings as possible. Get in touch with your "frightened" self.
- d. Silently shout "stop" or the strongest word you would use to startle yourself. The aim of this exercise is to capture your full attention.
- e. After the negative thought is stopped, counter it with an assertive statement. For example, you're in a chair, and this thought comes to your mind: "I'm afraid of girls. I'm afraid they think I'm stupid and ugly." After shouting the thought-stopping word loudly in your mind, replace it with "Girls are human beings, and they need other people, too. Some of them would probably like me if they got to know me." Use your own words and phrases.
- f. Continue until you have done this twenty to forty times. Keep practicing until your "cue" word interrupts negative thoughts each time they occur. This technique has proven successful in a number of research projects, so give it a fair chance.

3. BEHAVIORAL REHEARSAL

The idea of rehearsing assertive behavior is to make you more uninhibited and forthright in your actual conversations. Behavioral assertiveness training is usually done with a therapist or in a group; it's difficult to do by yourself. It might be done, however, with a cooperative and intelligent friend. First try to locate a local group or counselor who specializes in this problem. If none are available, then make an arrangement with a friend to work together.

a. Set aside forty to sixty minutes in a quiet environment.

b. Pose a problem. For example: discuss a complaint with your employer.

c. Your friend plays the role of the boss. Try to imagine your friend as that person, and say exactly what you really want to say. Your friend should try to imitate the boss in style and personality. Act stronger than you would if the situation were real. It works better if you overdramatize in the practice.

d. After five or ten minutes, reverse roles, and try to take your boss's viewpoint. Be as realistic as possible and as sympathetic and understanding of his position as you can. Try to understand what he must be thinking and what problems he has.

e. You may repeat this situation as many times as you like or go on to another when you feel you are ready.

f. You may have plenty of situations to practice. Here a few more suggestions:

- Politeness—practice saying "excuse me," "pardon me," etc.

- Pretend you're approaching someone at a party or at the office. How do you open the conversation? How do you continue it?

- Express your dissatisfaction at the poor service you have received in a restaurant, a department store, etc.

- Express your real opinions to another person. Don't stop to edit what you think.

- Cope with a rejection for a date, a job, etc.

Additional Thoughts

There is no way out. You have to face fears in order to grow. You can grow out of social anxieties, but not without risks. If you use the good nutritional formulas we have provided, you will be able to take risks and grow faster.

Nothing can make you progress more rapidly than mastering social skills such as manners, conversation, and confidence. Local colleges and some high schools have classes available. If there are none in your area, check with the regional or state psychological association or other referral sources.

Increased self-esteem and self-worth can only be brought about through your own efforts. When you do have a successful encounter, be sure you give yourself a pat on the back. If you deny credit to yourself where credit is due, then you rob yourself of another chance to grow.

You can learn a lot by observing others who handle social situations well. You must be your own therapist and know that changes only come about through repeated efforts. If you say to yourself, "I shouldn't have to do this," then check your attitude. You *do* have to do it—no one else will.

Nutritional Supplementation for Social Situations

One hour before entering a social situation that you expect will make you anxious, take the following supplements:

1. Thiamine, one (500 mg) tablet
2. Mintran (from Standard Process Labs, 2023 West Wisconsin Avenue, Milwaukee, Wisconsin 53233), three tablets
3. Choline, one (1,000 mg) tablet
4. Niacinamide, 250 mg

Additional aids:

1. Rescue, an herb preparation, 3 or 4 drops under the tongue for anxiety
2. Aspirin, 5 grains
3. Biotin, 1 mcg

PAST CRISES—RAPE, ROBBERY, ASSAULT, NATURAL DISASTERS

All crises have something in common—shock, intensity, and profound effect—but each one is also unique. The stresses they produce, however, cause psychological changes, which are similar in everyone. These common changes occur without regard to preexisting personality characteristics. In other words, no matter what a person was like before the trauma, he will undergo changes in response to it that are quite similar to those experienced by others who have had similar crises. The only thing different is that, depending on the personality dynamics, it may take a longer or lesser time to develop neurotic symptoms.

The personality's ability to recuperate from a disaster is not limitless. Human personalities can be fragmented so badly that in some cases they may never regenerate. Of those who do seem to adjust to their losses, no one recovers completely. Time by itself is a slow healer and often not a very good one. Many who remain untreated after traumas become worse rather than better with time. The effects on each individual can be great, and there is some evidence that the aftermath of trauma may continue on and become symptomatic in one's offspring, even those born years later (Rakoff 1966).

Although rape is not a communal disaster such as a major earthquake or tornado, its effects on the individual can be similar. Memories and images of the crime retain vividness years after the event. If the episode was severe enough, a person's life can be changed forever; elements of one's life are permanently altered. Images persist and so do the fears associated with the circumstances of the ordeal.

If the disaster was a tornado, for example, then fear is likely to be associated with winds and rain. From then on, whenever the traumatized person is exposed to wind or rain, excessive anxiety and fear are aroused. These exaggerated fears are recognized by the individual as irrational, but he can't avoid reacting. He may pace the floor or be unable to sleep when he sees storm clouds gathering, and in time his anxieties may even affect those around him.

Those who survive a disaster have had their illusion of invulnerability shattered. They now know, without question, that they are vulnerable to any new threat and may feel even more helpless than before. At night they often have terrifying dreams in which they struggle in a seemingly helpless situation, or sometimes they dream of their own death.

Many such persons become unreasonable in their requests for support. At the same time they may wonder if the support is genuine or simply given in response to their demands. This is often the case with any neurotic need for assurance. Since the support has to be dragged out of others, the individual cannot be sure it's given for the right reasons.

Intermixed with the need for loving support is the need for a focus for anger. Enraged at the assault on their person, victims want to have something or someone to take their anger out on. It's often difficult to restrain the seething anger that rages beneath the surface. Anger can also be an excellent coping mechanism with which to maintain some control over stormy feelings. However the anger manifests itself, interpersonal relationships are often impaired.

In disasters where others have died, there are usually additional feelings of guilt which must be dealt with. To have survived when others have died makes some victims feel (irrationally) that their life was purchased at the cost of others'. Perhaps, the survivor feels, he could have done more to save the others or perhaps he rightfully should have shared their fate. Feeling personally responsible for the outcome of the event can preoccupy the person's time and energy. It binds him firmly to the dead.

In most cases, if adjustments aren't made, the mental anguish starts to become physiological in the form of fatigue, gastrointestinal complaints, aches and pains, sluggishness, memory changes, confusion, disinterest in others, and even paranoid depression.

Studies on rape indicate that the initial symptoms after an attack include insomnia, depression, and school and/or work problems (Felice and Grant 1978). Fear, of course, was the first symptom: fear of leaving home, fear of strangers, and constant recurring nightmares. These fears were gradually discounted as the patients began to deny them. Patients would say they were no longer bothered, despite the fact they still had nightmares, insomnia, and the need to sleep with lights on.

Eventually these victims experienced the same physical symptoms as victims of other forms of disaster—headaches, abdominal pains, dizzy spells, etc. Psychological literature indicates that rape victims may suffer the same far-reaching adverse effects as those who survive natural disasters. For many, there is intense anger and bitterness, and the feeling of being violated and abused becomes virtually too much to bear. In many ways it parallels the feelings of Vietnam war veterans who suffer from posttrauma syndrome.

Not everyone falls apart after a disaster. Many adjust reasonably well and continue on much as they did prior to the crisis. Those who can't readjust usually seek some sort of help. Those who remain angry, resentful, and depressed and who can't or won't let go of their feelings need professional help.

POSTWAR DISASTER SYNDROME

Common symptoms were noted in veterans of the Vietnam War and the 1973 Yom Kippur War, all of whom were receiving medical psychiatric treatment (Borman 1986). In the Borman study, a group of such patients was compared with soldiers who had done no overseas service and with a second group of soldiers who had been used as support troops only. Each group was found to have about the same symptoms. Studies have shown that violence and drug abuse by soldiers in Vietnam correlated closely with preenlistment manifestations of such deviant behavior. This report by Borman suggests that vets who had a posttraumatic stress disorder did not necessarily develop it because of their experience in the war. That they may have had all the signs before they enlisted is not new information. The report indicates that severe stress may only make those with deviant behavior more conspicuous. In this case, we are not just dealing with depression and anxiety, we are dealing with a major personality disorder.

Help for Postdisaster (War, Rape, Assault) Victims

1.   If you're taking it pretty hard, or if it's been a long time since the crisis and you're still brooding about it, then self-help is not for you. If you haven't sought advice, then you should do so because your problem is just too much for one person to handle.
2.   Support groups are absolutely essential for this type of problem. You will benefit a great deal from the nutrients listed, but you also need some help from others.
3.   Medications can help relieve severe symptoms and may be used until you can gradually be weaned to the point of only needing nutritional supplements.
4.   Nutritional supplements:
   a.   Nutra-Homo, 1 tbs. 3 times daily
   b.   Niacinamide, 1,000 mg 3 times daily
   c.   See Chapter 14 for insomnia
   d.   Thiamine, 500 mg 3 times a day
   e.   Calcium lactate, 500 mg 3 times a day
   f.   Choline, 1000 mg 3 times a day

HOMOPHOBIA—FEAR OF HOMOSEXUALS

The fear of homosexuals seems to go back for centuries. It is strongly rooted in many religions, as some churches have condemned homosexuality as immoral and against God. Even in contemporary religious circles, it is considered by some to be sick, immoral, and antisocial. Until the mid 1970s, scarcely ten years ago, the medical profession considered homosexuality to be a severe emotional illness. In my own residency program, certain teachers expressed the opinion that homosexuality was a form of schizophrenia. But the pendulum always swings, and, at this writing, it is the "fear of homosexuals" that is now considered to be a "severe personality disturbance," damaging to both homosexuals and to society.

Part of the fear of homosexuality stems from the fear of its consequences on society, and some have considered it a threat to the very fabric of our culture. In the 1960s, homosexuals were rated the third most dangerous group in the United States, just behind communists and atheists. As late as 1983, a *Newsweek* survey indicated that only a third of the adults surveyed thought homosexuality was an acceptable alternative life-style.

Historically, gays have always existed on the fringes of society, partly due to revulsion at such practices as sadomasochism, promiscuity, cross-dressing, effeminacy, and passiveness. Added to this was the fear of homosexual teachers and youth leaders who occasionally molest youngsters, although the incidence of such cases is minuscule compared to that of parents who abuse their own children.

Homonegativism includes both a fear of the sexual connotations and a fear of the unknown. A lack of knowledge about or communication with homosexuals makes any experience with them fraught with uncertainty. It can be very anxiety-producing for a man, as an example, to relate to another particular man in any way contrary to what he has been taught is "normal," for such relating is thought to require a slightly different set of manners. Traditional male training and the behavior of animals seem to produce competitive behavior among males, a lack of submission, and a need for dominance. It is out of character for a male to be attracted to a male. Values are now being altered, and changes in what is considered acceptable often bring on irritation and anger. Repeated experiences in social situations with homosexuals will eventually create new social skills and ease the tensions for everyone.

Fear of Being Homosexual

Fear of homosexuals is not the same as being afraid that one is or might be a homosexual. The thought that one might be erotically aroused by a member of the same sex can cause acute anxiety or even panic. In a male there are all sorts of connotations: fear of submission, fear of failure as a man, loss of masculine power, etc.

Sometimes this homosexual panic is nonsexual in nature and really relates more to a fear of success. There is a symbolic transference of success fears to a fear of other men. First it is a fear of separation, of being too independent, and a fear of castrating others, a fear of helplessness which invites retaliation. The individual then surrenders to passivity; he relinquishes his goals and ambitions and thereby forfeits his masculinity. Taking the more feminine, submissive approach, he begins to suspect he might be homosexual.

Heterosexual men and women who are secure about their own sexual orientation and who have a firm gender identity are not threatened by homosexuals. Often the more macho a male is, the more threatened he is by gay men, and sometimes the only way he can feel safe is to assault a homosexual verbally or even physically. Physical abuse of gays has declined significantly in recent years, but there were times when brutalizing them was something of a sport —*fashionable and condoned by society.*

AIDS PHOBIA

Homophobia has currently all but been replaced by AIDS phobia, which is, of course, the fear of catching AIDS. Perhaps it would be better to say that AIDS phobia is an intensification of homophobia that has reached hysteria proportions. Early on, many public organizations received hundreds of calls from hysterical people, frightened that they might be exposing themselves to AIDS by mere social contact. Doctors and those in allied professions were not themselves immune from this hysteria, and panic in the medical profession peaked in 1984. Despite the preponderance of evidence that the disease cannot be spread through casual contact, doctors are still not presenting a united front; some continue to feel the evidence is inconclusive.

The public is even more unsettled and unsure about what to believe. According to a December 1986 *Los Angeles Times* poll, more than 50 percent of the respondents favored the quarantining of AIDS patients, and just as many favored a law making it a crime for AIDS sufferers to have sex with others. In the same pool, 48 percent said they would not like to have their child attend a school where a child with AIDS was enrolled. Since then, opinions have been modified by further education, but suspicion and fear still remain.

Insurance companies are concerned for another reason. The basis for their homophobia comes from facing the astronomical costs of AIDS care and treatment. The current cost for the treatment of one AIDS patient exceeds $140,000 a year. Faced with a disease that doubles its number of victims every year, they risk the loss of billions of dollars. Some insurance companies have reportedly resorted to rejecting applicants who live in known homosexual areas, especially if the person is male and unmarried.

The enormity of the situation has yet to be grasped. At this moment, the number of reported cases is doubling each year. Even though there has been a radical reduction in homosexual promiscuity, the number of cases continues to climb. The public has still not decided whether to empathize with AIDS patients or blame them because, even now, some homosexuals with AIDS are still found to knowingly infect others with the disease.

ARC—Sitting on a Time Bomb

Patients with AIDS-related complex (ARC) display greater stress levels than those with full-blown AIDS. They express high levels of uncertainty, for they feel that they are sitting on a virtual time bomb. Eventually, they will represent an enormous mental health problem because within a few years, ARC victims are expected to number in the millions. Over 180,000 now have this disease, and the growth rate is astronomical. ARC patients have the same anxieties as those who have been diagnosed with incurable cancer. They fear they will become burdens on others; they fear almost certain death, not to mention loss of mental capacity and disfigurement. Significantly higher levels of depression and anxiety are inevitable, as they face rejection and isolation. Many will have these fears realized, so such anxiety is unfortunately well founded.

AIDS Phobia Among Homosexuals

Among homosexuals, there is a group suffering from an exaggerated anxiety of contracting AIDS. These individuals check their temperature and search their body for blemishes daily. Worrying about AIDS becomes a preoccupation. Such patients begin to create in themselves symptoms of the disease—fatigue, sweating, difficulty with concentration. Their actions mimic the fear of syphilis (syphilophobia), or another disease, dysmorephobia, a fear of ugliness or disfigurement. This can gradually turn into complete hypochondria. Patients will appear in doctors' offices repeatedly seeking evaluations for AIDS, sometimes to the point of withdrawing from daily activity. Obsessed with their fears, they become profoundly disabled.

Doctors who treat AIDS patients have not escaped similar anxieties. Some develop anxiety reactions such as fear of death, nightmares, depression, AIDS-related contagion phobia, sex withdrawal, and general feelings of inadequacy. It is enormously taxing emotionally for doctors to see young, healthy patients wither and die, with no relief in sight. AIDS doctors are now experiencing combat fatigue which can last for years and is similar to posttrauma syndrome.

Overcoming AIDS Phobia

The first step is learning more about the problem, understanding that the infection is spread by sexual contact or injection of blood or contaminated blood products. For many, vulnerability to AIDS is very unlikely, but our knowledge of how to protect ourselves from the disease is still incomplete. For example, there is a lag time of several weeks between exposure to the AIDS virus (HTLV-III) and the formation of antibodies. During this time the infected person could pass undetected through standard tests for blood donations.

Tattooing, ear piercing, acupuncture, dental work, and any other procedure that requires needles should be done with great caution. All needles should be used only once, then destroyed. In the case of barbers and hairdressers, razors which might be contaminated with blood should be disposed of or thoroughly cleaned and disinfected. Cosmetologists, manicurists, pedicurists, or anyone who handles sharp instruments such as knives or scissors that could puncture the skin should make sure the tools are thoroughly disinfected. At the moment there is no evidence that the disease is being transmitted through such procedures, but all professionals should practice good hygiene and make scrupulous use of disinfectants.

Food service workers involved in the preparation or serving of food or beverages (cooks, caterers, servers, waiters, bartenders, airline attendants, etc.) should also exercise caution, although no evidence has so far emerged that the preparation or serving of food is a viable form of transmission. All food service workers should avoid injuring their hands, and any food contaminated with blood should be discarded. Anyone with open sores or weeping sores should refrain from direct contact with food intended for other people until healed. Sterilization, disinfection, and waste disposal information is now being circulated to health care providers.

The laundry and dishwashing cycles commonly used are generally adequate, and household bleach is a very effective germicide—1:10 to 1:100 dilution is effective. AIDS is not known to spread through the use of telephones, office equipment, toilets, showers, or water fountains. Any equipment contaminated by blood or bodily fluids should be cleaned with soap and water, then with 1:10 to 1:100 dilution of household bleach.

Patients with homophobia and AIDS phobia seem to respond well to antidepressant therapy. A dose of 150 mg of imipramine daily has produced successful results. Use the nutritional supplements suggested for posttraumatic stress (see p. 178).

WORRY

We all know what worry is, for we've all done it plenty of times, but how to describe it accurately is another matter. We could define it as a way of working out our problems, or as a tormentor that harasses us and gives us no peace of mind. Older literature has referred to it as "having cares," while newer authors say it's a low-grade fear, synonymous with anxiety. It has recognizable qualities, whether it's just enough to solve a problem, or intense enough to make us depressed, anxious, and unable to sleep. We all agree that it's not pleasant. A second important quality is that it is not a passive problem. We create worry ourselves at first, but later it may become a monster that takes us over and controls us in an obsessive way. A third quality is that worry represents a value judgment—the outcome of our worrying is important to us.

Worry—Threat of Loss

The benefit of worry is that it is usually painful, and pain is a strong motivator that forces us to take action. This means that, if we don't worry, the outcome could possibly go against us, and we may fail to get whatever it is we value. If we know we will succeed, we have a feeling of security and confidence. Not knowing for sure, we feel insecure and thus suffer anxiety, but the upshot is that we will probably end up working harder.

Worry—Care

While all worry is uncomfortable, there are degrees of discomfort. The more we feel we are running the show, the more chance there is that worry is a friend instead of an enemy. In business or sports, for example, worry produces results. Worrying the problem through is necessary, for it keeps our mind intensely focused on the problem, and that constant reality-testing helps us to cope with the situation until it's solved. When the problem is acute, such as in the case of a coach who faces a crucial football game, worry is part of the job. If the game is close, a coach will have about three and a half hours of intense worry—the kind that really keeps the adrenaline pumping! A good coach will worry, and the more he cares, the more intense his feelings will be.

In business we often have to wait for things to happen, and during this waiting period, we have time to worry about a problem, to recheck our plans and review our work. The same is true when we worry about relationships. Worry is a sign of concern.

Worry also serves as a way for people to readjust their minds to what is happening around them. It's a process by which they can prepare to tolerate the outcome of some pending event. If there is a danger of being hurt or disappointed, one can rehearse the event in his mind, visualizing what he would do under each possible set of circumstances, and how he would cope.

What to Do with Your Time—Worry

The next reason for people to worry has to do with the use of time. Eric Berne, in his book *Games People Play* (Grove Press, 1964), says that many people have trouble structuring time. We are all given sixteen hours a day in which to do *something*. Our bodies are built to keep us alert and awake during the daytime hours so we can fulfill our needs. Most animals require most of their waking hours to deal with matters of survival, but man has risen above this, and now finds that he has time to spare. Smart people fill their time wisely, but most of us don't. Either we were not taught by our parents how to use our time, or, even worse, we were taught unproductive ways of filling up idle hours. One of these "bad habits" passed on from one generation to the next is the fine art of worrying. Children of parents who worry a lot will tend to copy their role models, especially if the parents encourage them to. They solve their time-structuring problem (poorly)—worrying takes time. Now when they have spare time, they automatically turn on the worry machine and let it run for a while.

Worrying to Set Things Right

Another reason why people worry is to "set things right." If people have been embarrassed or slighted by another's insensitivity, they feel angry and resentful. In our mind, we create fantasies of recip- rocal rejection and conjure up ways to "teach the other person a lesson." In this way, we make things come out right. Making ration- alizing, self-righteous statements to ourselves can make us feel better. One of the major functions of this type of worry is to rewrite the script so that we can feel justified. *Self-righteousness is one of the major functions of worry.*

Worry—Control

The most important reason why we worry is to try to gain control over something we sense is out of our grasp. When we want things to turn out a particular way, and we need to prevent a bad outcome, we try to find new strategies that might give us better control. We search endlessly for more ways to manipulate circumstances, and we constantly reappraise the alternatives. Are there any we may have missed? What are the possible consequences if we fail? How terrible will life be without the one thing we think will bring us satisfaction? Overvaluing the object of desire in order to ensure its deliverance can set us up for catastrophe if we should fail to get it.

Worry—Pseudo-Control

Worry can also become a substitute for real control over a situation. If we are worried about a problem, we can convince ouselves we are exercising some control over it. This can even be carried so far as allowing ourselves to think that worry itself will magically be able to change things.

Worry—Hope

Worry is sometimes a way of fighting off feelings of helplessness and hopelessness. We are seeking hope in the face of uncertainty. With worry, we can prepare for the worst if it comes, but we can also hope for the best. With all the fears and anxieties of worry, there is also a strong element of hope, making worry a strange mixture of our most positive and negative thoughts. Without hope, we would not be worried—we would be in despair.

Worry—Obsessive Thoughts

Worry can also be a defense against the full onslaught of nervousness. Any repetitive action somehow buffers us against the pain of unrelenting fear and anxiety. Some people pace the floor, some sit in chairs and rock back and forth, some endlessly chew gum. Others indulge in excessive repetition; they run the same thoughts through their mind over and over again like a broken record. This is done deliberately to keep themselves distracted from their fears. The dullness of repetitive thinking is preferable to the experience of total fear.

When anxiety reaches the level of habit and progresses to the level of chronic discomfort, it becomes a disease. If the chain of thoughts and images becomes too emotional, worrying becomes less and less controllable and may become a compulsion. If we have no way of terminating it, it begins to cut into other parts of our lives and takes over. It can now emerge, at will, throughout the day, and we are helpless to stop it.

Worry Leads to More Worry

The problem with unchecked or uncontrolled ruminations is that they inevitably lead to more and more negative thoughts. Excessive negativism with its high emotional content sucks out all our energy and leaves us tired and spent. In susceptible individuals these endless thoughts may overstep into reality, as in cases of obsessive jealousy. A constant sense of threat—worry in its most extreme form—leads straight on to paranoia.

A major problem that accompanies excessive worry is insomnia. Once insomnia begins, so does the vicious cycle, for we are left tired the following day. Fatigue makes it harder to think straight, leading to increasingly poor decisions. And of course bad decisions cause more problems to worry about and more reasons not to sleep. Insomniacs who consult doctors usually say they just can't stop "thinking." They can't seem to turn their thoughts and images off.

There are some worries that are insidious. We misdefine our feelings as wants or needs, and yet what we're really experiencing is worry that has become out of control. Such feelings can escalate into extremes.

Reversing Worry

1. *Medication.* Antidepressants have been extremely valuable in reversing anxiety, even more than tranquilizers. Morbid worry should be treated only by a doctor. Self-help is not applicable here.

2. Nutritional supplements.

If depressed, tired, and worried, start with the following supplements:

- Tyrosine, two 500 mg tablets 3 times a day
- Phenylalanine, one 500 mg tablet 3 times a day
- Tryptophan, one 500 mg tablet 3 times a day
- Nutra-Homo, 1 tablespoon twice daily

Optional:

- Lecithin, two 1,200 mg capsules 3 times a day

3. Select a time of the day to worry—give yourself a half hour of time. All worries that occur during the day should be postponed until the preselected time.

4. During the worry period, concentrate on making it productive. Avoid self-righteousness—do not simply try to justify your actions or thoughts.

5. Write down your worries; work them out in writing. This will help you:

- Keep your problems in focus.
- See the worries more clearly.
- Reduce repetition.

6. Get in touch with your feelings. Watch your feelings. Learn to know when you are worried, and learn to recognize also when you are worrying unnecessarily.

7. Look at what it is you're worried about.

- Have you overvalued it?
- How much do you care about it really?
- Could you care less about it if you tried?
- Are you making too much of the consequences if you don't get what you want?
- Could you adapt to necessary changes more easily than you think?

- Will anyone really care about this in fifty years?
- Will *you* really care about this in twenty years?
- Do you cope better than you pretend to?
- Are you really as helpless as you think?
- If the worst happens, could you do something about it?

8.   Worry is fine if it's making you get things done. Has your worry become exaggerated and all-consuming?

9.   Repeat to yourself:

- Have I thought of all my alternatives? If the answer is yes, then you don't have to go over them again.
- Is there any new information I have to add to help the problem? If the answer is no, then you have no reason to start worrying again.
- Are there any circumstances I can control better now than I could before? If the answer is no, then stop worrying.
- There is no purpose to worry if I can't change things. Therefore, I will not worry. There is a saying that applies here—God help me change the things I can, and accept the things I can't. And have the wisdom to know the difference.

10.   Plan to keep a diary. Before you start:

- Estimate the amount of time you spend worrying each day.
- Estimate how tense your worries make you.
- Estimate how greatly they interfere with your happiness, progress, and success.

11.   Keep a diary for four weeks. You must persist for that long to notice any long-term benefit. Don't expect immediate relief. The techniques mentioned here have already proven themselves in research situations. Over 90 percent of those treated have been helped.

PART
3

CONQUERING THE COMMON FEARS

10

How to Conquer Fears in Business

Almost everyone in business experiences pressure. Those who can't take it usually get out or take jobs in lower-pressure areas. Some people, on the other hand, seem to thrive on tension and are well equipped to cope with it. This chapter addresses those who must face pressures but haven't yet learned how to deal with them effectively, as well as those who experience anxiety handling specific challenges such as public speaking.

FEAR OF SUCCESS

A fat person near his goal on a weight-loss program suddenly breaks his diet and starts to binge himself back up to obesity. An alcoholic, achieving recognition for his successful abstinence, unexpectedly falls off the wagon and disappoints everyone. A starlet on the verge of fame blows her big opportunity. Stories such as these are familiar and not uncommon, for fear of success strikes those striving in all areas of life.

Neurotic Anxiety and Success

Neurotic anxiety basically means using maladaptive coping techniques to control tension. There are better ways to handle stress

193

(relaxation, meditation, etc.), but the neurotic does not usually avail himself of positive methods because he is not fully aware of the extent of his anxiety. He only vaguely recognizes feelings of discomfort and does not see that his problem is really an overactive nervous system. Instead, he often jumps straight to the wrong conclusion, namely that a real and identifiable danger is the enemy. Such people seem to have a need to find some external cause for their discomfort; and when they do, they focus their fears on that object. It satisfies the need to know, found in all of us, and gives a focus for avoidance behavior. Once begun, unfortunately, the pattern usually continues. The feared object or event is a symbolic projection, a bogus enemy.

Freud's View

Freud and the psychoanalysts have had a field day with fear of success. It fits so perfectly into theories of unconscious forces at play. Many people apparently develop high levels of anxiety as they near their long-cherished goals. As their anxiety builds, they suddenly use their previous unsuccessful anxiety-releasing methods to cope with intolerable tension.

Since there is no real danger involved with being successful, the source of anxiety must be internal. It has to be an intrapsychic event. In the psychoanalytical concept, the danger originates in the feeling of being helpless or becoming too vulnerable in the new situation. Normally, anxiety develops when the person senses something bad is about to happen, but in the case of success anxieties, it develops on the brink of a breakthrough.

Psychoanalysts prefer to think of this anxiety as a displacement of unacceptable, sexual, aggressive urges. According to this theory, there develops an unconscious fear of castration should these urges become known to others. Fear of success, they say, is an oedipal dread of surpassing or castrating people (mother, father, or authority figures) who could initiate dreaded retaliation. To succeed is, in a sense, a highly aggressive act. To some, it signifies excessive competition, which is sure to be followed by a counterattack from others.

The more unimportant and undeserving a person feels, the greater his sense of helplessness. If he lacks self-confidence and self-esteem, then how could he ever be able to resist the retaliation of those who might be offended by his success? To display aggression is almost like throwing down the gauntlet to others. Fighting means being more independent and thus more alone. This can produce a *separation* fear, which is nearly universal. To become passive and fail is to reestablish dependency. It means, in essence, not to separate from others. And rather than bringing on retaliation, it invites sympathy and condolences and togetherness.

Success, whether a promotion or a graduation, is, in a sense, reaching a pinnacle of independence (separation), which places one at higher risk than ever before. If one lacks self-confidence, doubts arise as to whether success is worth the dangers. Maybe success will only generate problems and, eventually, failure. The public exposure will certainly initiate more circumstances in which higher levels of anxiety will have to be tolerated. Neurotics do not handle anxiety well to begin with, so what they are bringing into their life is more of what they wish to avoid—anxiety. By remaining in the background, they can maintain safety and not expose their weaknesses or inadequacies.

Other Reasons to Fear Success

The fear of being an impostor is very common among successful people, especially among intellectuals and scientists. To step back from the limelight is both prudent and respectable. When they do so, they are easily forgiven because they are no longer threatening the position of others. Though such persons may long for success, they justifiably fear it because they know they will become subject to unmerciful criticism by others who may be jealous. In these circles no one is allowed too much grandstanding—just quiet dignified respect.

Women are particularly vulnerable to success phobias, not instinctively but because of early training. Competition is played down in all areas of their lives, be it business, academic, marital, or maternal pursuits. Although it is socially acceptable for women to compete with each other for men, this should be done without involving overt aggressiveness. Even today, career ambition is less admired in women. It seems to arouse more animosity among both women and men than does ambition in a man, which is traditionally expected.

Because women are taught to be more self-sacrificing and passive than men, success can result in a "masculine image," which creates extra internal conflicts that must eventually be resolved. Success, by some definitions, is the equivalent of selfishness, as is power in all forms. All of this may be difficult to deal with. The autonomy that comes with success conflicts with roles in life that are more other-oriented, such as those of wife and mother. The possibility of surpassing both parents and one's husband can be an inhibiting concept.

Success can also be interpreted as a possible dissolution of self, a change in one's identity. Hardly anything will panic a person more than the threat of a major personality change. Expanding one's influence means gathering newer and better coping skills, and that requires a lot of work. Is it worth it? Success brings new demands and can threaten old familiar ways.

TREATMENT OF THE FEAR OF SUCCESS NUTRITIONALLY

1. Thiamine, 200 mg 3 times daily and at bedtime
2. Choline, 500 mg 3 times daily and at bedtime
3. Calcium lactate, 350 mg 3 times daily and at bedtime
4. Niacinamide, 1,000 mg B_6, 50 mg 3 times a day
5. Inositol, 500 mg 3 times a day
6. Lecithin, 1,200 mg 3 times a day and at bedtime
7. Magnesium orotate, 100 mg 3 times daily

The Failure Point

Review your past history. At what point do you seem to fail? For an obese person, there is usually a point at which he gets "stuck"— he reaches a certain weight, and he blows his diet. To succeed with these patients means controlling their anxiety as they approach their usual failure point. The same is true in fear of success. One must be very careful at this point not to miss a single nutritional supplement. It only takes a small amount of anxiety to destroy all progress. Until you are safely past your particular danger point, you will always be at risk. Be alert to this crisis point and religiously take your supplements as it draws near.

FEAR IN THE WORKPLACE—EVERYDAY FEARS AT WORK

Timid and nonassertive individuals often fail in their attempts to get what they want and are frequently treated unfairly. They are not able to take a stand, because they do not feel safe enough to express their real feelings. How this pattern develops is unclear. The possibilities range from genetics to environmental influences. Animal research has implicated both.

HOW SEVERE ARE YOUR FEARS AFFECTING YOUR CAREER?

	YES	NO
1. Have your fears had a major effect on your work performance?	_____	_____
2. Have your fears interfered with normal work in minor ways?	_____	_____
3. Have your fears been mild enough that they do not interfere with normal work?	_____	_____
4. Is your fear occasionally uncontrollable?	_____	_____

If you answered yes to three out of the four questions, then you can use the treatment that follows. But first go back through Chapter 4 and define your true goals as precisely as possible. A generalization such as "standing up to people" is too vague for this purpose, so be sure you clarify your specific desires in detail.

Exercise 1—Rehearse with a Helper to Increase Confrontational Skills

Rehearse with a partner, either a family member or friend, but choose someone with common sense and sensitivity. Your helper should not be afraid of confrontations.

1. Take your nutritional supplements an hour before you do the exercise.

2. Make up a list of situations that usually cause your anxiety.

A suggested list follows, but you may add situations of your own:

- Disagreeing with a friend over where to go on an evening out
- Refusing an unreasonable request
- Criticizing a friend whose habits are annoying
- Contradicting someone
- Questioning a fellow employee's activities
- Starting a conversation with a stranger

Make sure you have included as many real-life possibilities as you can think of, especially those which you find "sticky" or threatening. Your helper will, of course, play the role of the other person—parent, authority figure, employer, stranger, or friend.

3. Rearrange the list so the least anxiety-ridden encounters are at the top and the most troublesome are at the bottom of the list.

4. Take the first problem and rehearse the confrontation with your partner. Continue the discourse for at least five minutes, keeping the confrontation as lively as possible.

5. Stop and ask your friend for constructive criticism regarding the way you handled yourself.

6. Now reverse the roles and let your friend observe how each of you react in the same situation. If you feel anxious during this exchange, keep repeating it until you can experience it without fear.

7. If possible, use a tape recorder and review the conversation with your helper until you both agree that you are handling the situation satisfactorily.

8. After one problem is under control, go on to the next, using the same procedure in each instance. As soon as one situation becomes comfortable, continue on.

9.   When you feel you've made some substantial improvement, you can begin to be more assertive in your daily life, but do so cautiously at first. Save your first tries for reasonably safe situations, then gradually take on tougher problems.

Exercise 2—Rehearsal by Yourself

1.   Take your nutritional supplements one hour before beginning the exercise.

2.   Make up a list of situations that produce anxiety.

3.   Set a specific goal (I'm going to request a raise, I'm going to ask her for a date, etc.).

4.   Start with situation number one and go down the list. Practice using a tape recorder so you can speak out loud and play back your responses.

5.   Criticize yourself and speculate how you might improve.

6.   Be more aware of those around you who are comfortably assertive—how do they seem to do it?

7.   If you have a friend or acquaintance whose assertiveness you admire, ask him or her for advice.

8.   As you rehearse, be actively involved. Set up two chairs facing each other. Chair one is you, chair two is for the "other" person. Say what you want to say, then switch chairs and respond the way you think the other person would. Keep changing chairs and keep the conversation moving back and forth.

Nutritional Treatment

Use the same formula for fear of success with these modifications: Some people may be made jittery by inositol. You may wish to discontinue it altogether if it has this effect on you. Another variation is to take a 1,200 mg tablet of lecithin along with it. As I've mentioned, lecithin contains phosphorus, which is a stimulant. If either the inositol or the lecithin makes you edgy, you can try one last variation: Take 1,000 mg of choline (two 500 mg tablets) along with each dose of the inositol and lecithin.

One tablespoon of Nutra-Homo in the morning and at the end of the work day (around 5 P.M.) can also boost energy.

Tyrosine, one 500 mg tablet at 8 A.M., 11 A.M., and 4 P.M., is also helpful.

Phenylalanine, one 250 mg tablet on the same schedule, may also be beneficial. Glutamic acid, 500 mg, may be added along with the phenylalanine and tyrosine. Trial and error is the only real way to determine what's best suited to your own personal chemistry.

Refer to Chapter 3 on food and chemical allergies to see if they apply, for they may have a major influence on your mental strength and stability.

Nutrition on the Job

I have suggested a nutritional routine for those with generally high fear levels. If, however, you are anticipating an especially anxiety-producing situation, take an extra set of the vitamins one hour before your confrontation. It will not completely eliminate your anxiety, but it may give you up to 90 percent relief.

If you're a woman, remember that hormone balance is necessary for mental stability. If you're unsure about your homone levels, see your physician. Women who've undergone either surgical or natural menopause may require treatment. It also helps to exercise as often as possible. All this combined with the nutritional supplements should bring about changes rapidly.

Rehearsal Between Exercises

Rehearsal of confrontational material between exercises helps pro-long the effectiveness of the treatment. To go over and rehash the feared experience and any changes made during the treatment will make the sessions successful. This helps prevent a phenomenon known as resensitization (rekindled fears), which may take place between each confrontation.

Those who had rapid and more intense heart rates during exposure to feared objects did not do as well as those with a slower heart rate (Sartory and Rochman 1982). Magnesium orotate, 50 mg, and niacinamide or B_6 tend to slow the heart, so there is less palpitation. You may add the magnesium to your supplements, especially if you know you have mitral valve prolapse.

Exercise 3—Arm Muscle Tightening

If you have ever seen or heard of a muscle-building technique called "dynamite tension," then you will know immediately how to do this exercise. Place your hands together about twelve inches in front of your mid-chest area, and pit the strength of one arm against the other. Keep the hands firmly locked together and muster up all the strength you can, while tensing any other muscles you wish in your shoulders, chest, neck, or abdomen. It helps to take a deep breath first, then push your hands and arms together as hard as possible. Continue for five or ten seconds or until you feel tired. Then let go. Let the tension drain out of your body, and say to yourself, "Warm, warm, warm." Usually, by then, you will start to feel very warm and relaxed all over. After doing this exercise two to four times, you should feel quite loose and reasonably relaxed, ready for a confrontation.

Exercise 4—Paradoxical Intention

Review the material on Paradoxical Intention on p. 81. This technique is also useful in confrontations.

FEAR OF LOSING CONTROL OF AGGRESSIVE IMPULSES

In one study, a group of agoraphobic males had rarely experienced panic attacks (Hafner 1986). Instead, they feared a loss of control over aggressive impulses to harm themselves or others, either physically or verbally. Internal aggression can sometimes lead to physical harm if a person reacts by leaping from a bridge or in front of a moving vehicle. Physical and verbal aggression toward others was found most likely to occur in crowded or confined places.

The agoraphobic men in this research program were treated with behavioral therapy. The before-and-after hostility tests showed that the level of hostility and the number of objects to which it was directed (people, events, places, etc.) dropped significantly twelve months after treatment. While in therapy, these patients were also more able to face their self-destructive impulses.

Some men seem to seek the title "Master of the World." While they might consciously dismiss this as a simple childhood dream, they feel chronic anger when coping with the challenges arising from their quest for environmental control. Extremely aggressive businessmen, those classified as "Type A" personalities, often end up with heart attacks. Treatment to prevent early cardiac problems includes learning better coping skills.

Treating these disorders with relaxation techniques (Hart 1984) has proved beneficial. Behavioral therapy can alter the self-destructive Type-A behavior. Learning muscle-tension awareness as well as techniques to reduce general tensions is useful for Type-A individuals, who usually have poor awareness of their bodily changes during times of anger and frustration. When they are taught to make a self-analysis and then to use reversal techniques, their behavior can change for the better.

Aggressive behavior, or the suppression of aggressive impulses, can play a big role in anxiety, and anxiety plays a significant role in mental illness. Even though this book deals more with fear than with anger, the latter can often be a form of disguised fear.

TREATMENT FOR AGGRESSIVE IMPULSES
THAT RELATE TO FEAR

1. Use the relaxation techniques in Chapter 4.

2. You can buy Standard Process Labs niacinamide, 50 mg tablets, and B_6, 10 mg capsules, and use 4 to 8 when angry, for quick results.

3. An alternative method is to use four 500 mg niacinamide tablets along with one 50 mg B_6 tablet when you get angry, and repeat every

2 to 4 hours if the situation gets worse. This dose may be doubled when necessary.

4. 400 mg tablets of Miltown (meprobamate), a prescription drug, is also useful during episodes of anger.

5. Propranolol tablets have been used very successfully for chronic anger—again, they must be prescribed by a physician.

6. If your anger is severe, don't rely on self-help alone. It's possible to make improvements on your own, but don't deprive yourself of the benefits of professional treatment if such assistance is needed.

PHONOPHOBIA

Taking a bath, crossing the street, answering the phone, or making a call are all commonplace events for most people. But for some, the simple act of using the phone can be a major challenge.

An example is George Brown, a midlevel executive. He spends his busy day communicating easily with others both above and below him on the corporate ladder. There is no question as to his competence as a manager; he is an experienced and high-energy worker, known to be levelheaded and serious by nature. He does, however, have one secret—a personal flaw, which he hides from his fellow workers. George is afraid to use the telephone. Even the thought of making a phone call will reduce him to a bundle of nerves.

Brown does make phone calls, of course, but not without considerable discomfort. He usually puts his calls off as long as he can; often panicky and flustered, palms sweating and heart racing, he picks up the phone. His voice is pinched and strained, so he keeps his conversations brief. He uses various devices to hide his unnatural voice.

George makes all his calls while in his private office with the doors closed so no one will overhear. It is virtually impossible for him to telephone in front of another person. Since everything has to be "just right" before George can make a call, and business situations do not always permit him to arrange his necessary conditions, George loses a lot of valuable time preparing for his calls and gathering the courage to make them.

There are certain types of calls, of course, that no one likes to make, such as calling in sick or delivering bad news. But some people are so sensitive that they break out in a sweat just dialing information. There are a number of explanations as to why this happens. It has been suggested that a phone conversation is less controllable than a face-to-face encounter, and like fearful flyers who panic at the thought of not being in control, phonophobics freeze at the thought of taking a verbal "plunge." It's not unusual for such persons to make their calls at a time when they are relatively sure the other person will not be in. It's a game they play with themselves to prove that they really can make phone calls. The element of the unknown plays a role here, for a conversation with a voice only, especially if it belongs to a relative stranger, can produce varying degrees of discomfort.

This uneasiness in handling a phone task can be made more palatable by changing the environment in which the calls are made. Here are some suggestions:

1. Stand up while making calls. Standing increases the sense of power. Walking around a little during the call also dissipates tension and creates some distraction.

2. Push-button phones are easier to use and may lessen apprehension.

3. Prepare ahead for the call by making a list of all the subjects to be covered. In this way there is less uncertainty and more control over the conversation.

4. Open windows or turn on more lights in the room; expand your environment. This reduces the element of feeling alone or helpless and provides a figurative "escape" hatch (in case you need to dive out the window).

5. Go through a brief rehearsal prior to the call. Enact the whole dialogue, taking both sides of the conversation. Make it a pleasant, congenial, and friendly encounter.

6. Listen to relaxation tapes.

7. Use the relaxation techniques listed in Chapter 4.

8. Save all your phone calls for one particular time of day, then take these supplements an hour before you start the phoning:

- Thiamine, 250 mg
- Calcium lactate, 500 mg
- Choline, 1,500 mg
- Niacinamide, 500 mg
- Biotin, 1,000 mcg
- B_6, 25 mg
- Pantothenic acid, 1,000 mg

If you find this technique successful, but you want to be independent of the supplements, cut the amount each week by 10 percent, and you may find yourself self-sufficient in as little as 10 weeks.

STAGE FRIGHT

Stage fright can affect anyone—amateur or veteran performer. When it strikes, its symptoms include a pounding heart, knees that tremble, sweating hands, failing memory, dizziness, and nausea. Some of our most famous entertainers still confess to stage fright in spite of experience and success. Even days before a performance, an artist may suffer nightmares, headaches, or anxiety attacks. Some cope by taking alcohol, tranquilizers, or street drugs.

Performance Anxiety

Another name for this might be fear of failure, and it could be described as an obsession about "measuring up" to real or imagined standards. This obsession interferes with concentration on the work itself and robs the performer of the energy that should be going into preparation and performance. It depletes him of the vitality necessary for the actual event, thus at times becoming a self-fulfilling prophecy.

This nervous energy can, however, add to a performance by providing an extra edge. Every performance is, in a certain sense, a test, and one that is judged by others. The result can be standing ovations or public humiliation, from the sublime to the ridiculous, and each performance has a bearing on future survival. For those who make their living in the limelight, everything is *truly* on the line. Perhaps the magic "something" that sparks so many performances is a need for survival as much as it is the need for approval.

While many performers can force themselves to function in spite of paralyzing performance anxiety, others cannot. Racked with insomnia, tension, and panic, their tempers flare, and they earn the reputation of "temperamental star," which doesn't help them land future work.

At some point, in a good performance, all this energy is released, and the show "goes on," as they say. Adrenaline in the bloodstream, which, prior to the show, caused nothing but anxiety, now serves to keep the artist alert and focused. It gives him an extra "rush"— just the thing needed for a smashing show.

Expectations as Problems

A loss of self-esteem can often bring on these anxieties. Being out of a job, for example, can result in depression and insecurity. Every job interview soon becomes equated with survival. If one feels that there should come a point in life when one can stop proving oneself, stop competing, then it's a shock to discover that this seldom really happens. It's a fact of life that no matter how high you go, you will still have to keep producing, keep proving yourself, and keep selling yourself.

We are all sensitive to the expectations of others, but if we are too sensitive, we tend to develop an exaggerated sense of responsibility, and we believe that others expect nothing less than perfection from us. We may feel every mistake will be forever held against us and that only a flawless performance is acceptable. Holding ourselves up against such impossible expectations is not only unrealistic but dangerous. The anxiety it causes can bring about the very thing we fear, namely, more mistakes and decreased productivity.

Tranquilizers and sedatives only mask the problem; while they may reduce our anxiety, they do nothing to increase our performance. It becomes so easy to depend on them, just as some rely on alcohol. And like alcohol, a ubiquitous hazard in the entertainment industry, sedatives can become addictive and cause careers to suffer.

Treating Stage Fright

There are some time-honored ways to handle performance anxiety. Some of them are scoffed at, and yet they proved themselves useful long before the advent of drugs or modern therapy.

1. One of these "devices" is superstition—the simple faith that a good-luck charm will carry one through. For some, it's a piece of jewelry or a particular garment. Frequently, faith in an object actually lowers the anxiety and fear levels, and things consequently go better. Superstition may seem out of place in modern society, but placebo effects can work just as well as drugs and psychotherapy, and without the consequences of addiction or expense. Faith and superstition, if not carried to extremes, can be viable techniques for self-control.

There is currently a resurgence of respect for "animal" instinct—knowing something on a gut level, without hard evidence. In both the business and scientific worlds, a sense of keen intuition is considered valuable. Faith and superstition are extensions of this undefinable but well-regarded ability.

2. Ceremony can be another valuable tool. Taking a bath, then going through a particular dressing ritual, is, for some, soothing and reassuring and a great anxiety reducer. When he always follows such a routine, whether it be complicated or simple, an actor, for example, may feel more in control. If there is an especially satisfying way of preparing for a performance or event, then it would be wise to make that routine a habit, especially during times of stress.

3. Meditation or relaxation exercises are also good ways to handle anxieties. These techniques should be practiced until they can be done rapidly and successfully. Once mastered, they can be used to tackle a variety of problems. Eastern religions have used meditation for centuries, so proof of its value is well established. Relaxation tapes are a shortcut technique that some have found useful.

4. Watch your diet. Cigarettes, caffeine, sugar, and alcohol all increase anxiety. Sugar and alcohol do this during the withdrawal process, and caffeine and nicotine directly affect the adrenal glands. An anxious person needs more adrenaline like Custer needed more Indians.

5. Constructive activities can also help control anxiety. Movement per se dissipates tensions. If you lived on a farm, you could chop wood, but city dwellers can jog, do aerobics, or go for a brisk walk.

6. Just being outside is sometimes very soothing. Going to a garden, a park, or walking by the ocean can quickly put you into a better state of mind. I once worked at Patton State Mental Hospital in San Bernardino, California. At that time, the hospital was connected to a farm, and the inmates were able to grow the food on their own. Along with providing a sense of self-sufficiency, it also put them in touch with the earth. In a very literal sense, they became grounded. The most disturbed patients were placed on the farm, where they worked in the soil or around animals, and it calmed them immeasurably. Nature is perhaps the best tranquilizer in the world, for it connects us with our roots and with the universe.

7. Monitor your conversations and thoughts and do not dwell on catastrophes. You have enough problems without adding the burden of endless self-condemnations. If you catch yourself creating negative thoughts, bring them to a quick halt and then find something more positive to think about. The one thing you definitely can control is what you think.

8. Do not berate yourself for being nervous. It goes with the territory. If you are going to do something as exciting, glamorous, and interesting as being on stage or in front of an audience, you're going to have to survive the natural fears of self-confrontation. In a sense, an audience is like a giant mirror in which you can see every imperfection. You will never be satisfied with what you see (few artists are); but if you get a favorable reaction, if your audience likes what they see, that's the most important thing. It's okay to respect their opinion, too, as well as your own, and enjoy the applause.

9. Propranolol was being used as a cardiac medication when it was discovered to also have a sedative effect. It's sometimes been used to calm stage fright because it blocks the body's beta-receptors and other places in the nervous system where adrenaline affects the cells. There is one problem with this drug, however—it does have side effects. Many people report feeling "strange" and not quite normal. Others develop low blood pressure as well as other symptoms. Nevertheless, in some research projects it has benefited the user.

NUTRITIONAL TREATMENT OF STAGE FRIGHT

Take the following nutritional supplements one hour before the performance:

- Thiamine, 500 mg
- Calcium lactate, 1,000 mg
- Choline, 1,000 mg
- Niacinamide, 500 mg
- B_6, 50 mg
- Biotin, 2,000 mcg
- Aspirin, 5 grains
- Pantothenic acid, 1,000 mg
- Folic acid, 800 mcg (take 4 of these tablets)

11

How to Conquer the Fear of Going to School and Teenage Fears

Is School Refusal Rational?

As a parent, you may not fully realize that the school you are sending your child to is not quite the same as when you were a kid. Back in the "good ole days," the most serious disciplinary problems were talking in class, teasing, cutting, and pushing and shoving. All that may have seemed a bit hard to handle then, but it does not compare with what many kids have to face today. Drug and alcohol abuse, assault, rape, pregnancy, suicide, sexual permissiveness, and now the threat of AIDS are common and very real problems faced by children of the 1980s. School-related anxiety today may be more warranted now than ever before; in some cases it may be a survival response.

The Young Child

A mild fear of going to school is almost universal. Most parents understand this and try to provide reassurances. Some may even visit the school a couple of times to allow the child time to adapt. Most children need a little extra help during this period of transition; it's an occasion of initial separation for many. Even if they have been accustomed to staying with relatives and sitters, the security of exclusive attention is no longer guaranteed, and now the child must learn to share. How prone a child is to developing an overwhelming fear of school depends on both genetic constitution and home environment.

Surprisingly, many fearful students come from stable families, although others are, as expected, the products of turbulent households. If parents have been overly protective, the child will require more reassurance and adjustment time. If he is already vulnerable, fears may be intensified. Family problems may or may not play a role, depending on the child. What we do know for certain is that fear in childhood is common, and there are those who have inherited a special sensitivity or what's been described as a "readiness and reason to fear."

School is a whole new ball game for most kids. There are definite pressures and increased expectations. Teachers are often insensitive to susceptible children, unintentionally setting up awkward situations that lead to discomfort or even embarrassment. They may ask inappropriate questions in front of the class or be unreasonably punitive. Antagonistic teachers can set off these phobias or make them worse in their initial stages.

Over half of all school-phobic children begin to experience anxiety after changing schools, although these phobias are not as common as once thought. The most severe forms develop in about one child in a thousand, with moderate cases a little more prevalent.

A mother's social behavior is a powerful impact on a child's normal or deviant behavior. Without realizing what she's doing, a mother may actually be reinforcing a child's incorrect responses. It has been found that by correcting the mother's actions, the child's behavior can often be improved (Wohler and Winkler 1965).

Children who develop severe cases of this phobia are often overly worried about normal events such as menstruation. They worry about their parents when they are in school, and frequently complain about relationships with other children. They sometimes report being bullied or teased and may be afraid of their teachers. They are frequently self-conscious individuals, overly concerned about their own behavior.

CHILDREN WHO ARE UNUSUALLY ANXIOUS

Physical signs that a child is overly fearful of going to school are usually present, and a parent should pay particular attention to these unconscious behaviors.

1. Unusually stiff posture
2. Fearful facial expressions
3. Problems with inattention
4. Avoids eye contact
5. Contorts lips
6. Lips tremble
7. Stuttering
8. Inability to sit still
9. Sucks or chews on objects
10. Fingers in mouth
11. Licks lips frequently
12. Nail biting
13. Does not answer questions
14. Whispers or speaks softly
15. Whining voice
16. Frequently uses "afraid," "scared," or other similar words
17. Often wants to leave parties or social situations
18. Uses physical complaint words frequently: stomachache, headache, earache, etc.

THE FIRST SIGN OF SCHOOL REFUSAL

Psychologists have a number of theories to explain the refusal to go to school. Some think it's a fear of separation from the mother, or perhaps a fear of disappointing one's parents. Whatever the case, these children are often shocked to find adults cynical about their problems.

Children frequently use ill health as an excuse for avoiding school and will manifest such symptoms as diarrhea, stomach pains, sweating, trembling, and faintness. They may feign a cold or cough or ear trouble. Once they are assured of staying home, they usually begin to get better, especially when school hours are over. While at school, they may complain to others about a fear of fainting or vomiting in front of others.

Are Parents Rearing Kids Right?

Some studies have indicated that parents who overprotect their children without displaying personal warmth create psychological conditions in the child that can lead to the later development of all types of phobias, including an excessive fear of school (W. A. Arrindell, P. M. G. Emmelkamp, E. Brilman, and A. Monsina, 1983). Being overprotective, while at the same time showing signs of rejecting the child, sets up conflicting signals that confuse and undermine psychological stability. Keeping a child physically safe is not a satisfactory replacement for caring and affection. It behooves the parent to check his behavior toward the child to see if perhaps he is substituting overprotectiveness for warmth and closeness. It has been suggested that the consistent sending of double messages can precipitate mental illness in most genetically vulnerable individuals.

Social phobics (those who are unduly uncomfortable around others) frequently complain of having been overprotected by their parents. Such behavior often results in a restricted environment, a lack of opportunity for normal social development, and extended dependence. Lack of training in social skills can also be damaging to the child; in later years the patient's unrecognized sense of social incompetency produces a continuous level of anxiety that can lead to school phobias among other disorders.

It should be clearly pointed out that most studies are based on recollections of how the adult phobic perceives his early childhood, and there is no verification as to accuracy. In other words, the results of an interaction may stem just as much from the child's perception of what's happening as from what actually takes place. Sensitive children can and often do distort reality.

Depression and Anxiety

The term *school phobias* actually covers quite a broad area and includes a collection of neurotic disorders associated with a grave reluctance to attend school. Truancy accounts for from 10 to 30 percent of the school refusers, while physical and mental disorders are factors in a smaller proportion. It has been found that those with major psychological imbalances form the largest group and tend to belong to two subgroups: those with predominant depression and those with predominant anxiety.

PHYSICAL CAUSES OF SCHOOL PHOBIAS

School phobias often originate after a period of physical or mental stress, either perceived or actual. For example, sudden acute mononucleosis may leave the patient debilitated and vulnerable. With the advent of newer therapies, many children who would have died from cancer continue to live with chronic malignancies; school phobias often develop within this group. Drugs, too, may alter biochemistry, as was the case of one group of young patients being treated for Tourette's syndrome. Fifteen developed school refusal after being treated with a drug called haloperidol (Mikkelson, Detior, and Cohen 1981). Decreasing the dose or eliminating the drug caused reversal of that phobia. Such an occurrence indicates that some people have a biochemistry programmed for phobias and may exhibit symptoms the moment their system is thrown out of balance.

Family doctors and pediatricians should be aware of triggers that set off school phobias. It has been suggested by various experts that alert practitioners could prevent many of these phobias if they caught and treated them at an early stage.

TRUANCY

Truancy should be suspected in anyone who shows reluctance to go to school. Up to a third of all alleged phobics are not really avoiding school because of a phobia. Chronic truancy is not to be confused with school phobia, for there are a number of characteristics that separate them.

The Truant Child	*The School-Phobic Child*
1. Uses strategies to stay away from school	1. Stays home or in safe place such as library
2. Spends time alone or with another truant	2. Spends time alone or with the family
3. Is often associated with delinquent behavior	3. No delinquent behavior
4. Poor grades	4. Good grades
5. No exaggerated complaints about ill health	5. Frequent complaints of stomach disorders, insomnia, nausea, etc.

A Way to Tell

If you suspect that your child is afraid to go to school, have him or her take the following tests. If the child is too young to respond in writing, you can read the statements and record the answers.

TEST 1—HOW DOES YOUR CHILD GET ALONG WITH TEACHERS?

If a child gets along poorly with his or her teachers, then a phobia may be developing.

Young Student's Rating Scale

	YES	NO
1. I can talk to my teacher easily.	_____	_____
2. She nags and scolds me.	_____	_____
3. She is very friendly	_____	_____
4. She insists I do things her way.	_____	_____
5. She praises me when I have done well.	_____	_____
6. She punishes me unfairly.	_____	_____

	YES	NO
7. She helps me with school work when I don't understand something.	_____	_____
8. She embarrasses me in front of others.	_____	_____
9. She teaches me things I want to learn.	_____	_____
10. She appears disappointed in me.	_____	_____
11. She says nice things to me.	_____	_____
12. She makes me get permission for everything.	_____	_____
13. She enjoys having me in her class.	_____	_____
14. She expects too much from me.	_____	_____
15. She encourages me often.	_____	_____
16. She tells me she doesn't like me.	_____	_____

Scoring

The even-numbered statements indicate a negative feeling about the teacher. A score of over five indicates problems. The odd-numbered statements indicate a good relationship with the teacher—an unlikely situation in a school phobic.

TEST 2—HOW DOES YOUR CHILD GET ALONG WITH OTHER CHILDREN?

This is another major factor in the development of school phobias.

Getting Along with Other Children

	YES	NO
1. My friends stick up for me.	_____	_____
2. Children around me are too bossy.	_____	_____
3. My friends make me laugh.	_____	_____

	YES	NO
4. Children around me are jealous of me.	_____	_____
5. My friends feel worried when I have a bad day.	_____	_____
6. The others make fun of me.	_____	_____
7. Other children play fair.	_____	_____
8. Kids are always getting upset with me.	_____	_____
9. Children around me usually smile.	_____	_____
10. Kids always seem to pick on me.	_____	_____
11. Kids always invite me to join in their games.	_____	_____
12. I always get the blame for everything.	_____	_____
13. My friends do nice things for me.	_____	_____
14. Other children give me dirty looks.	_____	_____
15. People are so friendly to me.	_____	_____

Yes scores on the odd numbers indicate good social adjustment. Five or more yes's on the even-numbered statements indicate problems with other children and possibly a tendency toward school phobia.

TEST 3—HOW MUCH ANXIETY DOES YOUR CHILD HAVE?

High anxiety levels can contribute to the development of school phobia.

Child's General Anxiety Level

	YES	NO
1. I'm afraid of thunderstorms.	_____	_____
2. I get nightmares.	_____	_____

	YES	NO
3. I hate to hear my parents argue.	___	___
4. I hate for my parents to criticize me.	___	___
5. I'm afraid of the dark.	___	___
6. Spooky things scare me.	___	___
7. I'm afraid of getting into a fight.	___	___
8. My heart sometimes beats fast.	___	___
9. My feelings get hurt easily.	___	___
10. I get tired a lot.	___	___
11. Strange-looking people scare me.	___	___
12. Playing rough games scares me.	___	___
13. Making mistakes upsets me a lot.	___	___
14. I'm afraid I might look foolish.	___	___
15. I get frightened taking a test.	___	___
16. I'm afraid the teacher will call on me in class.	___	___
17. I don't like people to look at me.	___	___
18. I feel awful when I get punished.	___	___
19. I can't stand getting a shot from a nurse.	___	___
20. Spiders and bees scare me.	___	___

This test is just an indication of general anxiety. The number of fears not only relates to abnormalities, but also to age groups. In other words, three- to six-year-olds are in a high-anxiety period and would probably have a number of yes answers. On the other hand, eight- to nine-year-olds with more than ten yes answers may have a problem.

HOW TO HELP YOUR CHILD GET OVER HIS FEAR OF GOING TO SCHOOL

Drugs

In 1969 Robimer and Klein ("Imipramine Treatment of School Phobias") used an antidepressant to treat twenty-eight children who
wished to avoid school; twenty-four out of the twenty-eight were
able to return, and there was a general improvement in behavior of
85 percent of that group. It was thought at the time that the patients
were being treated for separation anxiety, but, true or false, the
improvement was very significant. The most important point here
is that the children responded to the antidepressants. This type of
knowledge leads us toward various theories on how to successfully
apply nutritional supplements.

Nutritional Supplements

Nutritional supplements have already proven to be quite effective
in changing children's behavior. The problem, of course, is getting
kids to take the supplements on a regular basis. You can nag the
older ones, but little ones must receive their supplements from their
parents, and this can put an extra burden on an already busy mom
or dad.

The amino acid analysis is the superior approach because it gives
accurate, personalized information. If it's not possible, then here are
some suggestions. Listed below are the most useful supplements in
descending order of importance. Start at the top and work down,
adding new ones if your child tolerates it. After you do see results,
you must continue supplementing or the symptoms will return. It
usually takes more than a year of supplementation before you can
safely begin to decrease the doses.

NUTRA-HOMO POWDER

In small children over five, use ¼ to ½ teaspoon of powder. Ages
six to ten years, use ½ to one teaspoonful twice daily. In older

children, follow the directions on the can, which is generally one tablespoonful two times daily.

I prefer this supplement for a starter because it is in powder form and can easily be taken in juice, so there's no problem with swallowing pills. Its flavor can easily be disguised in tomato or vegetable juice. The most important reason for using this product is that it is about the most complete supplement around. Its nutrients, vitamins, and amino acids combine to make a complete nutritional package. Consult with your physician before adding any of the following ingredients.

KYOLIC GARLIC OIL

This is available as a capsule or liquid. Naturally, I prefer the liquid because the child can absorb the larger doses without having to swallow a pill. Small children could take one to three capsules a day, and older children six to eight. Adults need twelve to start with. Many people will not be able to tolerate so much garlic in the beginning; they may start at the lower end of the scale and work up gradually.

Why are we suggesting garlic for young children? Because it supplies thiamine in its purest form. Large doses of thiamine are required to calm the hypothalamus, which, in turn, quiets the neurological system that creates anxiety.

If you fail to get your child to accept garlic, don't despair. Just concentrate on the Nutra-Homo, and keep trying to introduce the garlic every so often because it is a valuable addition to the program and will prove well worth the effort.

Note: Garlic is slow to show its effects and sometimes must be taken for as long as a year, but the results are generally long lasting. If you are troubled by the garlic's odor, you may wish to deodorize it with some liquid chlorophyll. If you are unsuccessful in getting your child to take either of the two items, you may try a liquid B-complex formula, which can be found in most health food stores. Although it won't be as effective as the Nutra-Homo or the garlic, it will be of some value.

LIQUID CHOLINE

Why did I mention liquid choline instead of lecithin? The answer is that choline alone is a tranquilizer, while lecithin can be very stimulating because of its phosphorus content. Phosphorus is a stimulant. You will need to experiment with different doses. For small children, 50 mg twice daily is useful, for larger children seven to nine years old 100 mg twice daily, and for teenagers, 500–1,000 mg is recommended. I have suggested moderate doses, but they may be increased in some cases.

INOSITOL

Choline should always be balanced properly with inositol, so add about half as much as your dose of choline.

NIACINAMIDE-B_6

Standard Process Labs manufactures an excellent combination capsule with a 50 to 10 ratio of niacinamide to B_6. The capsules can be pulled apart and the powder combined with other powders in juice. Young children may start with half a capsule twice daily, and those over ten can take a full capsule three times daily. I suggest conservative doses here, but you could try more; adults often use two 500 mg capsules of niacinamide, three or four times daily, with a high degree of safety. Experience with depressed patients and alcoholics has shown that thousands of milligrams daily have been relatively safe.

VITAMIN B_6

Small doses of B_6 are safe and are useful to the general metabolism. However, if the Nutra-Homo has been successfully taken, B_6 will not be necessary. Paradoxyl-5-phosphate is the preferred form of the vitamin and comes in capsule form. It's easy to open the capsule and put half the amount in food, twice daily. It usually comes in 50 mg doses, and young children should only have a quarter of this amount.

For depression I recommend two amino acids, tyrosine and phenylalanine. A dose of 100 mg of tyrosine twice daily and 50 mg of phenylalanine twice daily is recommended for younger children, while teenagers can take one 500 mg tablets three times daily. Middle-range children should use a half tablet of tyrosine twice a day. Phenylalanine should be given in doses half that of tyrosine.

Amino Acid Analysis

In Chapter 2, I discussed the amino-acid analysis test. The information gained from this test has turned around many a young life. It requires the help of a physician and is important because it can pinpoint exact underlying causes of many emotional disorders. The percentage of improvement using this therapy is well over 90 percent for each patient. Behavioral problems generally respond quite nicely. If the problem is severe, this type of treatment can save the day. In Chapter 18 you will find the address of the Atron Company, which will provide you with a list of doctors who do amino-acid analysis. This approach is, by far, the best because it tells you exactly what will help the child.

Desensitization

I have defined and discussed desensitization in other parts of the book, especially in Chapter 5, so I will only briefly discuss it here. If you wish to read about it in more depth, turn back to p. 115. Basically, desensitization means teaching the child to face his fears gradually over a period of weeks. For thirty minutes, twice each week, you should expose your child to increasingly greater amounts of anxiety, until he is able to handle significant contact with the object of his fear.

Desensitization, with or without other techniques, has reduced school phobias, horse phobias, fear of heights, fear of darkness, fear of automobiles, fear of bathrooms, fear of making mistakes, fear of water, and fear of hospitals, as well as stuttering and the fears of reading, loud voices, and tests. Desensitization can be achieved by gradually facing the actual feared object whether in reality or in the child's imagination. It has been found, however, that facing the actual object rather than fantasizing about it produces much faster results. I'll give you two examples of ways to work.

Developing Your Hierarchy

Set up a graduated hierarchy similar to the two suggested ones below. Progress in about eight steps starting from what the child can actually do now to the final desired result; each step will be slightly more difficult than the one before.

Work with the child, helping him or her imagine the scenes in your list. Plan to spend thirty minutes, two to four times a week, working together. Usually improvements become visible within one or two weeks, but continue until you are satisfied.

Since each step is harder than the one before, you'll need to teach your child how to cope with his fears by using an "anxiety antagonistic response." In a nutshell, that means when the child complains of anxiety or nervousness, you'll teach him how to use his coping technique.

The best method for a child is to teach him to experience a pleasant scene in his imagination. Tailor the scene to his particular needs, and ask him to conjure up the most pleasant vision possible, such as something involving Christmas or Disneyland. Or you may try scenes from his favorite stories, using heroes from movies, books, or newspapers (Batman, Superman, Supergirl, etc.). How does your child see himself in the scene? As Superman? Or his sidekick? What is each one doing? The important thing is to experiment with different scenes until you think you have determined which one really gets his attention and holds his interest. Once that's accomplished, your child will have the best possible tool for coping with anxiety. In the future, as he goes through the steps of his hierarchy, he will learn to turn to this fantasy scene every time he feels discomfort.

It's always helpful when children see others in the presence of the thing they fear; people learn from observing those around them. Have you ever wondered how an animal is taught to dive off a high tower into a tank of water? It's done by letting the novice watch other more experienced animals perform the trick. The fine art of imitation of course applies to humans as well.

Always give the child the nutritional formula one hour before doing any of these exercises.

HIERARCHY NO. 1—IMAGINATION

Place a comfortable chair in a darkened room. Have the child sit down and get totally relaxed. Make sure he's prepared to imagine the scenes.

1. The mother angrily shakes the child awake and demands he get ready for school.

2. All through breakfast she lectures him about going to school; both parents are critical of his actions.

3. He's now on his way to school (by car, bus, or walking); and as he comes within a block of the school, he wonders what will happen when he gets there. Now the school is just around the corner. Now he can see it. Finally he stands directly in front of the building.

4. He enters the school, and all the kids stare, then begin to snicker. They act as though he is strange, as if he doesn't belong there. They say cruel things.

5. The teacher makes him go directly to the front of the class and stand in front of all the other children. The other kids laugh and make fun while the teacher announces to the class that he is stupid.

6. The teacher then asks him questions, but he's too scared to answer. He's frightened and wants to leave but the teacher refuses to allow him to sit down. She says he's going to have to stay in front of the class until he gets the right answers to her questions. She glares at him hatefully.

7. All of the kids talk among themselves, and he overhears some saying how stupid, how crazy, how ugly he is.

8. The teacher says that since he didn't answer her questions, he'll have to take a special test. Everyone laughs.

Have the child imagine each scene as vividly as possible in order to create a maximum amount of anxiety. Desensitization is the process of arousing anxieties that can be brought out and eventually dissipated. If the nutritional supplements are used correctly, they will keep the anxiety at a level that your child can tolerate while doing the exercise.

As the child experiences each scene, have him rate his level of anxiety:

- Not scared
- A little scared
- More than a little scared
- Really scared
- Too scared to go on

If a child should become too frightened to continue, stop the exercise until he regains a state of relaxation before moving on. In therapy it's possible to do one to three scenes in a twenty- or thirty-minute session. With the proper use of nutritional supplements, it's possible to do five or more scary scenes each session.

HIERARCHY NO. 2—REAL EXPOSURE TO SCHOOL

I have provided a suggested hierarchy to follow in order to prepare your child to face his school-related fears. Be sure he or she takes the correct nutritional supplements one hour before any of these sessions. Refer to the advice given on pp. 219–221 to ascertain the correct supplements for your child's age group. You should have a nutritionist's approval before using the supplements.

Now, instruct your child to do the following:

1. Get up, take your books out, get dressed, eat breakfast, and go outside. Be sure you're as ready as possible. Play it for real, and pretend you're going all the way.

2. Go through step 1 again, but this time walk several blocks toward the school. Pretend as much as you can, and convince yourself that this is the honest-to-goodness, real thing.

3. Go through step 1 another time; now walk all the way to the front door of the school. Arrive late so there won't be other children outside.

4. Go through steps 1 to 3 once more, and this time go through the halls of the school. Plan a time when everyone is in class, so the halls will be deserted.

5. Go to school while classes are changing and the halls are crowded with children. Say hello to some of the kids.

6. Make arrangements with the school ahead of time to attend class for just one hour.

7. Make arrangements to attend three classes in a row.

8. Arrange to spend one full day at school.

9. Arrange to spend three days in school.

10. Arrange to spend one week in school.

Note

- Be persistent and keep to your schedule.
- If you become too frightened at any step along the way, slip back to the level you can cope with, and begin again from there. Everybody has backslides. It's normal. Don't beat yourself over it.
- My hierarchy is just an example for you to work from. Create your own on the chart below.

PERSONAL HIERARCHY

Step 1 _____

Step 2 _____

Step 3 _____

Step 4 _____

Step 5 _____

Step 6 _____

Step 7 _____

Step 8 _____

Step 9 _____

Step 10 _____

Hierarchical treatments are rather old-fashioned, but I have included them because they work. Many people have conquered phobias using this technique, and it's always helpful to include multiple methods of treatment in any program because, as I keep emphasizing, each person is unique.

WHAT HAPPENS TO PEOPLE WHO AVOID SCHOOL?

What happens later on in life to children who avoid school? Studies are contradictory. Some show that most patients with school phobias go on to lead normal productive lives, while others indicate just the opposite, with a predominant number of patients suffering from adult fears that inhibit their potential. Consequently, adequate treatment of underlying problems is more important than merely returning the child to school. Most children go through phases where they will be fearful and cautious, and some will develop a fear of a specific item or place, but these anxieties usually diminish with time, both in intensity and frequency.

Those who do return to school are not always able to achieve their full potential. Even in school they fail to receive much benefit. It seems that whether a student returns to school or not has little to do with future career performance (Bakes and Willis 1979). Getting students to return seems superfluous to some researchers since it appears that their future is less affected by school attendance than by underlying instabilities. [In one three-year follow-up of a group of psychiatric inpatients, a third showed no improvement, and remained emotionally and socially impaired (Berg and Butler 1974). Another third had moderate improvement, and the final third were completely or almost completely recovered. Emotional symptoms tended to persist in patients with a chronic history of them (Berg and Fielding 1978), and even therapy showed little long-term effect.]

TEENAGERS

If you're an unusually sensitive, lonely, or insecure teenager or think that you might be, take this test and see how you fare.

Test for Teenagers

	YES	NO
1. I can't do things as easily as others.		
2. I worry about what people think of me.		
3. I worry too much.		
4. I am always nervous.		
5. I never seem to do things right.		
6. I'm always tired.		
7. My feelings get hurt easily.		

	YES	NO
8. I have trouble going to sleep.		
9. My mouth is dry. It's hard to swallow.		
10. I often regret things that I've done.		
11. I worry about what's going to happen to me.		
12. I don't like to talk in front of a roomful of people.		
13. I can't keep my mind on anything for very long.		
14. Others do not like the way I do things.		
15. I worry about my schoolwork.		
16. Most people are happier than I am.		
17. I get nervous when things don't go right.		
18. It's hard to make up my mind.		
19. When I go to bed I start to worry.		
20. I feel lonely a lot.		
21. I don't like others to look directly at me.		
22. My stomach bothers me a lot.		
23. I guess you could say I'm afraid of a lot of things.		
24. At times I get so nervous I feel like screaming.		

Ten or more yes answers indicate a higher than normal anxiety level. Eighteen or more yes's indicate severe anxiety.

You now have some idea about your level of anxiety, and we'll deal with that in a minute. For the moment let's measure how depressed you are, because depression and anxiety together can deal a double whammy both to your life and to your future.

Depression List

	YES	NO

1. My moods change often. I can get high, then very low. I'm on an emotional roller coaster. _____ _____

2. It's easy for me to cry. I can cry over any little thing, sometimes for no reason. _____ _____

3. I feel people don't really care about me. I feel that people don't want me. _____ _____

4. I don't like myself. I wish I were different. I don't do things right. I'm not happy with me. _____ _____

5. I think about "ending it all" a lot of the time. I'm not sure I wouldn't do it under the right circumstances. _____ _____

6. I'm bored with the world. What's the use? I feel empty. I don't care about anything anymore. _____ _____

7. I'm tired a lot. I just don't seem to have enough energy. At times I feel exhausted. _____ _____

8. I want to sleep, but I can't. I wish I could sleep more soundly, because I don't wake up rested. _____ _____

9. I seem to catch everything. I'm always sick. I don't think I'm very healthy. _____ _____

10. My stomach bothers me a lot, and it seems like my bowels aren't right. _____ _____

11. I'm on edge, I have no patience with people anymore. I snap at the slightest thing. _____ _____

12. Sometimes things don't seem quite real. All of a sudden everything feels strange. _____ _____

If you answered the test honestly, and four of the first six answers were yes, then you should make an appointment to see a therapist; you are probably more depressed than you realize. If you answered yes to two or less of the statements 1–6 and yes on four or more of the statements 7–12, then you are depressed enough to need to take action to change things.

Depressed children, in addition to being gloomy and tearful, often express feelings of being unloved as well as feeling isolated and alone. They perceive themselves as unloved whether they are or not.

By now you should have a more precise idea of just how depressed and anxious you are. If you're above average in these areas, you probably will want to change. Let's make one more quick analysis before we discuss what to do about your problems. Let's try to decide where you think your anxiety is coming from.

Fill in the questionnaire. I have—

1. A fear of criticism   _____
2. A fear of disappointing others   _____
3. A fear of failure   _____
4. A fear of embarrassment   _____
5. Too much parent pressure   _____
6. Too much school pressure   _____
7. Too much pressure in (fill in)   _____

_____

_____

I hope this gives you a clearer idea of where your problems lie and just how much you are affected. The good news is that gaining such knowledge is half the battle, so you're already ahead.

Doing Something About It

It's important to recognize that it's not stress that does people in, it's how we react to the stress. Since we all encounter stress throughout our lifetime, it is necessary for us to learn how best to cope.

This process is a major part of growing up, with emphasis on the word *growth*. Growth means becoming stronger and bigger and more competent, and it is an integral part of life. One of the fastest ways to encourage growth is to face your fears—avoidance only reaffirms our weakness. When we avoid our fears we avoid growth. In a nutshell: No growth = weakness; growth = strength.

Get Acquainted with Your Enemy

It always surprises me how many people are not in touch with their feelings. People will simply say they feel "bad," instead of saying, "I feel anxious," or "I feel anxious and depressed." Not really knowing and recognizing when you are anxious prevents you from doing anything constructive, thus your anxiety continues on. When you allow your anxiety to remain, you begin avoiding things; and when you avoid things, you don't grow; and when you don't grow, you don't become strong enough to get what you want and need. For that reason it's very important that you go to the trouble of being absolutely sure you recognize anxiety in yourself in order to be better in touch with your feelings. Only then can you take action.

You should know now that you are really the only one who can determine when you're anxious, and you alone are responsible for dealing with it. If you don't accept the responsibility for learning how to recognize anxiety and how to cope with it, then it's going to persist, and that means you are in for a lot of pain, for anxiety hurts like hell.

But for every dilemma, there is an answer. There are, of course, drugs which are effective but, as you have read elsewhere in the book, they have serious drawbacks. While drugs may initially reduce anxiety, they don't seem to have any long-term benefits. Sooner or later you must be taken off them, and unless you've made significant progress during the interim, the anxiety will return then, often stronger than before.

Nutritional supplements, on the other hand, can be used in such a way that they can relieve you of much of your anxiety without interfering with growth. In order to take your supplements correctly, you may need to make adjustments, and it might be wise to seek a nutritionist's advice and help during this period. At the same time you use these supplements, you should also take advantage of the coping devices that will help effect a lasting cure.

Nutritional Treatment for Teenage Anxiety

1. For the limited budget:
   B_1, one 500 mg tablet, 3 times a day
   Calcium lactate, one 350 mg tablet, 3 times a day and at bedtime
   Choline, one 1,000 mg tablet, 3 times a day and at bedtime
   Multivitamin, one tablet, twice a day
2. Other supplements that could be added:
   Niacinamide, one 500 mg tablet, 3 times a day and at bedtime
   Biotin, one 1,000 mcg tablet, 3 times a day and at bedtime
   Tryptophan, one 500 mg tablet, 3 times a day and at bedtime
   B_6, one 50 mg tablet, 3 times a day
3. If depression is a problem, the following may be added:
   Tyrosine, one 500 mg tablet, 3 times a day
   Phenylalanine, one 250 mg tablet, 3 times a day
   Magnesium, one 100 mg tablet, 3 times a day

Coping Mechanisms

1. Take your supplements on a regular basis, but on days when you expect special problems, time the nearest dose so that it is taken an hour before the extra stress.

2. Remember that coffee, diet colas, recreational drugs, cigarettes, and alcohol all undermine the effects of the supplements. Either eliminate these "blockers" or cut way down on them and increase your nutritional supplements to four times a day.

3. Refer to Chapter 4: Paradoxical Intention is a quick, easy-to-learn technique that effectively dissipates anxiety. Practice it conscientiously for seven days, and it will be your friend for life.

4. See page 201 for the coping technique of pressing your hands in front of your chest. It's easy to do, and it works quickly.

5. Relaxation tapes are extremely useful. Just put one in a Walkman and play it when you are facing a problem. If you listen to these tapes two or three times a day on a regular basis, you will probably begin to notice a steadily increasing sense of calmness.

6. Physical exercise is also an excellent tension reliever, if the exercise is intense enough to give you a real workout. For example, a leisurely ride on an exercycle for thirty minutes is not as effective as three to four minutes of intense cycling, followed by a rest, then three to four more minutes, followed by a final set.

FEAR OF EXAMS

Do you believe any of these things?

- I don't need to take exams.
- Exams aren't fair anyway.
- They don't really test your intelligence.

If you do, then whether you have admitted it to yourself or not, you are definitely afraid of exams. Does it make any difference if you try to correct this fear? One research group (Deffenbacher and Kemper 1974) reported significant improvement in grade point average when test anxiety in sixth-grade students was successfully treated with desensitization. Doing better in school counts for a lot, but relief from the intense pressure as one nears exam time is also important. What can you do to make things easier on yourself?

Getting Better Grades

Improving school performance comes down to two things (not counting being diligent about homework): controlling anxiety and developing better ways to handle tests. In fact, just learning how to increase control during exams reduces anxiety in well over 50 percent of all cases.

Take a course at your local college on how to take exams, and learn how to master specific coping techniques.

TAKING THE EXAM

1. Never walk out on an exam.
2. Present better work.
3. Spend some time, maybe ten minutes, just planning.

4. Determine the best order in which to answer questions.
5. Answer all the easy questions first.
6. Answer pet subjects early on.
7. Figure out the more difficult questions next.
8. Answer those questions you're unsure about last. Try making an educated guess.

NUTRITION AND EXAMS

After you have worked out the best nutritional formula to decrease anxiety, take that formula 90 minutes before the test. Just before entering the exam room, use your best anxiety coping device from the Coping Mechanisms list on page 232 and repeat it during the exam whenever you feel yourself becoming tense.

CAUTION

The best and safest approach in applying nutritional therapy to youngsters under 12 is to seek out a knowledgeable therapist. Lists of organizations and therapists are given in Chapter 18 and the Appendix. The Atron Company also has a list of pediatricians who utilize nutritional methods in the treatment of fears.

12

How to Conquer Fear of the Dentist

EVERYONE'S FEAR

Are you afraid of the dentist? Don't be ashamed to admit it—you're not alone. That particular anxiety is one of the most widespread forms of fear in everyday life and the most common problem faced by dentists today. But it's not just a problem of modern-day medicine; it appears to have been with us since the days when dentists sedated their patients with a swig of whiskey. Dental journals since the turn of the century have included articles on the dentist's role in trying to control his patients' anxieties.

Normal apprehension about dental treatment is not the same as being clinically disabled. Says one such patient, "My body reacted violently as I sat down in the dentist's chair. My heart was going crazy, my hands trembled, and my clothes were soaked. I felt like a coward, but I was ashamed to admit my fears, and I couldn't leave. I felt the doctor and his staff were secretly laughing at me. They *knew*."

This patient, like another 11 to 18 million Americans with dental phobias, finds it literally unbearable to see a dentist. One study found that about 6 percent of the U.S. population suffers from dental phobias to the point where they incur significant health problems (Friedman and Feldman 1958). The situation, of course, is severely compounded when these individuals finally do seek help because by then there is usually so much repair work needed that they truly face a painful ordeal.

Dental Anxiety

Dental anxiety ranges from the mild uneasiness experienced by most of us to acute anxiety attacks. It has been said that fear of dentistry may actually have a different quality to it than other phobias. Even so-called "fearless" patients do not display complete comfort during all dental procedures, so in a sense this could be called a true form of anticipatory anxiety, making total removal of fear virtually impossible.

Fear of the dentist varies from person to person. A few individuals literally fear the possibility of death, but these cases are extreme. Others fear facing an injection in the sensitive regions of the mouth. The fear of drilling brings dread to many, and just the sound of the drill can make many hearts skip a beat. Others fear the unknown, which is probably related to lack of control—an uncomfortable sensation under any circumstance.

Dental Pain

Fear of pain, however, is usually the most severe apprehension experienced by those with dental phobias. Although such individuals demonstrated no greater sensitivity to pain than a comparable group of nonphobics, a difference was noted in their tolerance to pain. Phobic patients showed higher anxiety levels and were overly reactive to dental paraphernalia, which could obviously translate into a more pronounced reaction to dental pain. Dental phobics often lack confidence in themselves and in their ability to cope with discomfort. They feel they are not going to be able to handle pain when it occurs, and they anticipate failure.

Dental fear is thought to be the most common cause for canceled appointments and is a major problem faced by dentists in routine practice. This phenomenon can, of course, be made worse by the way the dentist handles his patients. A callous practitioner can do much to strengthen the myth, and even sensitive dentists sometimes inadvertently reinforce the preprogrammed fears. For example, when patients get nervous, a caring dentist may stop and reassure them and hand out "rewards" to young children who cooperate. Studies have shown that both of these actions, far from being helpful, tend to reinforce the fear of dental pain.

Dentists, on first seeing a patient, must decide whether his or her fear is normal or abnormal. The question is, Will the fear respond to reason? If not, then it is apparently beyond voluntary control and must be considered pathological.

Psychology of Dental Fear

If dentistry is stressful for patients, it also poses difficulties for dentists. Cases have been reported where practicing dentists actually became phobic about practicing dentistry (Marks and Christopher 1979). Apparently this condition can manifest itself as a part of a burnout syndrome. Chronic stress produces a loss of job satisfaction and eventually causes fatigue and depression, resulting in a genuine aversion to the job.

It's often been stated in scientific literature that early adverse dental experiences are responsible for setting up a phobia. Other authors, however, have found that just as many people who did not develop phobias suffered dental trauma at a tender age (Klepac and Dowling 1982). It appears to take more than a single bad experience to produce the disorder and has more to do with response to the experience. Psychoanalysts have been quick to attach hidden meanings to dental fears such as the famous oedipal complex, fear of punishment, fear of authority figures, symbolic hate, etc. But much more likely, they are simply the result of a vulnerable person undergoing phobic learning by the classical, Pavlovian, conditioned reflex.

Dental Fear Test

If you are wondering whether or not you need help with this problem, take the following test:

I fear:	Mildly	Moderately	Severely
1. Open wounds	_____	_____	_____
2. Strange places	_____	_____	_____

I fear:	Mildly	Moderately	Severely
3. Pain	_____	_____	_____
4. Dentists	_____	_____	_____
5. Needles around the mouth	_____	_____	_____
6. Strangers	_____	_____	_____
7. Authoritative people	_____	_____	_____
8. Fast heartbeats	_____	_____	_____
9. Losing self-control	_____	_____	_____
10. Blood	_____	_____	_____
11. Having a tooth pulled	_____	_____	_____
12. Having a dentist working on my mouth	_____	_____	_____
13. Enclosed places	_____	_____	_____
14. Fainting	_____	_____	_____
15. Looking foolish	_____	_____	_____
16. Dental office smells	_____	_____	_____
17. Noisy dental drills	_____	_____	_____
18. Bright lights	_____	_____	_____
19. Suffocating	_____	_____	_____
20. Dental office waiting rooms	_____	_____	_____
21. Being unable to move	_____	_____	_____

I fear:	Mildly	Moderately	Severely
22. Difficulty in breathing	————	————	————
23. Dizziness	————	————	————
24. Dry mouth	————	————	————
25. Numbness in the mouth	————	————	————

Scoring the Test

Obviously, if most of your check marks are in the far right column, then you probably suffer from excessive dental fear. For solutions to this common disorder, read further.

TREATMENT

Administering an elaborate and time-consuming fear-reduction procedure is not necessary for most patients, but a fearful person needs more than mere determination to enable him to visit a dentist. The goal of most treatments is to reduce fear substantially, although total elimination of all fear is unrealistic. The accessible goal, therefore, is to reduce the level of fear to the point where a patient can go for the necessary treatment and, while undergoing procedures, suffer as little pain as possible.

The Dentist

An individual with a strong fear of dentists needs to be selective in his choice of practitioners. He requires a dentist who will understand his fears and help assure him that they can be dealt with. Some dentists are able to provide comforting assurance that allows the patient to gain confidence. Such a doctor could begin with a minimally aversive treatment. Finding a compassionate practitioner can often be accomplished by talking to friends and relatives, or by contacting the dental association in your area.

Some dentists prescribe medications to presedate the patient before he even comes to the office, while others use acupuncture or hypnosis. Both of these approaches are time-consuming but are well worth the trouble, especially if the patient is not going to avail himself of dental care any other way.

Control Your Thoughts

It's necessary to control one's thoughts prior to going to the dentist, in the reception room, and during treatment. Studies have shown that patients who think positively about dental treatment undergo less stress and less pain during the procedure (Richardson and Kelinknecht 1984). Those with catastrophically negative thoughts generally suffer accordingly. It has been found that negative thoughts are a major contributor to nervousness, and thus become a self-fulfilling prophecy (Last and Blanchard 1982).

The best approach is to allow yourself only positive thoughts from the time you leave the house until the time you return. Since you are dealing with a fear that tends to escalate the longer you have to wait, try to arrange to be seen as soon as you arrive at the office. This tactic is useful for another reason also—you will need to time your nutritional supplements. Take them approximately one to one and a half hours before the dental work begins, so that you can benefit from their maximum calming effect.

Thought Stopping

You will, of course, be constantly tempted to go back to your old ways. You'll literally *crave* old negative thoughts. It's a bad habit that must be broken. Once you start to give in, just a little bit, you'll soon be back to where you started. If you catch yourself thinking negative thoughts, you must quickly change them into positive ones.

How do you make the transition? It can best be done with a "thought-stopping" word or phrase, strongly expressed (mentally) such as "Stop it!" "Drop it," or "Knock it off." Virtually shout those orders to yourself immediately and sternly, in such a way that shocks you enough to turn your thinking around. You may have to repeat the process several times to be effective. If done properly, however, it *will* stop the negative thoughts. If you have difficulty concentrating, substitute thoughts about what you're doing at that moment or focus on what's going on around you.

Nutritional Supplementation

These should be taken one to one and a half hours before seeing the dentist. It would be wise to get his approval first.

1. Calcium lactate, three 365 mg tablets, for mild to moderate fears; this may be all that is necessary.
2. Extra helpers for greater fears:
   - Thiamine, one 500 mg tablet
   - Choline, three 500 mg tablets
   - Niacinamide, one 500 mg tablet
3. Additions for stronger fear levels:
   - Mintran, three tablets
   - Aspirin (five grains), one tablet
   - Tryptophan, one 500 mg tablet

An additional amino acid, D-phenylalanine, may also be taken for pain control. Take a 500 mg tablet both before you go and after you return from seeing the dentist.

If you decide to use nutritional supplements, you may combine them with any medication you receive, although you should always check with your dentist and let him or her know what you're doing. A dentist might opt for a shortcut and prescribe tranquilizers to deal with the situation. However, medication has its drawbacks:

- Many people object to the idea of a "pill for all occasions."
- The dentist may not want the patient medicated when he comes to the office.
- There may be side effects or other reasons why the patient cannot or should not engage in drug therapy.

Coping

Another useful technique is Paradoxical Intention. You will find this technique described on p. 81. It also works extremely well with the nutritional supplements. An additional technique you might want to try is using relaxation tapes. You could listen to one on the way to the dentist's office, and also in the waiting area, using a Walkman.

By now you should be familiar with the concept of desensitization as a gradual way to face your fears. It can either be done through imagery or real-life exposure. The reason you need to face your fears, even though they may be well controlled for a period of time by nutritional supplements, is that desensitization is the only way you will ever eliminate fear on a permanent basis.

Self-Help

EXERCISE NO. 1—DESENSITIZING THROUGH IMAGERY

1. Write out your ten worst situations hierarchy, or use the one suggested.

2. Write each hierarchy item on a three-by-five-inch note card.

3. Take your nutritional supplements one hour before the treatment session.

4. Achieve muscle relaxation or use a relaxation tape for a few minutes prior to your session, if you feel you need it. See Chapter 4: Relaxation is not essential for desensitization; use it only if you wish.

5. When thoroughly relaxed, pick up the first card and begin visualization for a thirty-second period. (You may use a timer, although it is not necessary.)

6. Stop visualization when the thirty seconds are up.

7. Stop visualization if any anxiety is experienced, and start the muscle relaxation procedure again.

8. Try to revisualize the scene and keep on repeating this procedure until you can visualize without any anxiety—now you can advance to the next card.

9. Continue on until all of the cards have been used.

10. How often should you practice? As often as you like, but at least a minimum of twice a week for six weeks.

Begin with the scene that causes the least anxiety and slowly work up to the one that causes maximum anxiety. Imagine the first scene. Repeated presentations of this scene will extinguish the associated anxiety. This process is continued on down the hierarchy until none of the scenes provokes distress. At this point, one is said to be deconditioned, and the effect should carry over to real-life situations.

A reclining chair puts you in an excellent position for desensitization. Imagine a scene, gradually working the period of time from thirty seconds to three minutes, then relax for one minute, then reimagine the same scene for three minutes, then relax again for one minute. You can use cards to remind yourself of each scene. If there is no anxiety, go on to the next. In thirty minutes, you should be able to do three scenes; however, with nutritional supplements, you may be able to do more than three in one session.

SUGGESTED HIERARCHY

1. Sitting at home thinking about tomorrow's dental appointment.
2. Driving to the dentist's office.
3. Waiting in the waiting room.
4. Sitting in the dental chair.
5. Having a dental prophylaxis (teeth being cleaned with a rubber cup in dental handpiece).
6. Having a dental probe scrape along your teeth.
7. Having a topical anesthetic placed on the gums.
8. Having the slow-speed drill scraping over a tooth (finishing burr).
9. Hearing the "whine" of the air-rotor close by.
10. Receiving an injection around an upper molar.

EXERCISE NO. 2—DESENSITIZING BY REAL EXPOSURE TO DENTIST'S OFFICE

Here's a self-help method that will enable you to desensitize yourself to dental visits. Choose a friend as a support person—though you can do this solo. Your support person should be someone who understands your fears and is willing to help you overcome them.

1. With support person, walk in and out of the dentist's office.

2. With support person, sit in the waiting room for two to five minutes.

3. With support person, sit in the waiting room for fifteen minutes.

4. Make an appointment with your dentist just to talk to him for a short while. Tell him your problem and explain that you are trying to desensitize yourself. Ask for his cooperation.

5. With support person nearby, sit in the dental chair for five to ten minutes without the dentist present, then leave.

6. With support person nearby, sit in the dental chair for ten to twenty minutes without the dentist in attendance, then leave.

7. With support person, make an appointment with the dentist to do a small amount of work, such as X rays or a cleaning.

8. With support person, make a longer appointment with the dentist, fifteen to twenty minutes, to do a small filling.

9. Without support person, make a longer appointment with the dentist, perhaps for two or three fillings.

Make sure your dentist is someone with whom you feel comfortable and in whom you can develop a trust; he or she should share your desire to overcome your dental fears.

CHILDREN AND DENTAL FEARS

Smaller children ages three to five are at the peak of their vulnerability to fear. Almost anything can unbalance them; strange places and unfamiliar people can be stressful and upsetting. Anxiety toward a dentist and his personnel is as normal in children as in adults, but it usually occurs on a more intense level. Ignoring these fears or negating them will only force them "underground" and cause them to reappear in some other form of misbehavior. It has been found that giving a frightened child a toy or gum as a bribe to "be good" will serve to reinforce rather than reduce the phobia.

Will a Parent's Presence Help the Fears?

Yes and no. If a parent has had a close warm relationship with the child, his or her presence may have a strong influence on the youngster's sense of security and thus increase his ability to cope.

Reports from some researchers, however, do not show a significant difference in child behavior as a result of the presence or absence of a mother during dental procedures. In some cases, the anxiety of the mother is strongly reflected in the child, and the dentist needs to be aware of this. Parents who openly express fear of the dentist and specific dental procedures in front of their children are sometimes asked to wait outside. Such mothers may move nervously in the chair, hide their eyes, make exaggerated facial signs of fear, or emit fearful sounds, all in the child's presence. Needless to say, such behavior doesn't provide much moral support!

Children over five seem to be significantly less affected than those who are younger. They appear to be more cooperative and less anxious with or without a parent's presence. It appears that fears are overcome through growth, added experience, and improved skills and self-confidence.

Helping Children Overcome the Fear of Dentists

Simple methods are not too complicated for preschool children to respond to. They can be taught to relax and breathe deeply or to use some other coping device. Go through the processes listed below, then after each procedure, ask the child to repeat it. Make the experience like a game and be as playful as possible. You may notice that the child is better at one technique than another; if so, concentrate on that one when he visits the dentist.

Teaching the Child to Cope

1. Refer to the section on relaxation in Chapter 4 (p. 83). With a little patience, children can be taught how to relax themselves. If they practice a few times, they can usually get quite good at it.

2. Refer to the breathing exercises in Chapter 4 (pp. 84-88). Show the child how it's done and assist him in doing each exercise correctly. Use several different practice sessions until he can do it without your help.

3. Ask the child to describe to you the most pleasant scene he can imagine. Keep working with him until you are sure it really is the best he can come up with and gives him a truly good feeling. It can be a favorite location, a favorite character (cartoon or real), or a favorite situation. Have him experience it in his imagination with eyes closed. This exercise and the one that follows have been found in many studies to be excellent coping techniques for children.

4. Practice "self-talk." "I am calm, everything is nice." "I will be all right in just a little while." "Everything is going to be okay." Let the child choose his own words if those phrases don't appeal to him or don't seem to be the way he or she would word such thoughts. Again, keep working with the child until you are sure you've come up with the best words and phrases possible.

Once a child learns coping devices, he should choose one or two he can do well enough to relieve anxiety during a visit to the dentist.

5. After each practice session, describe to the child what is going to happen.

- Describe the basic procedures he is going to experience.
- Describe the typical physical sensations. Relabel negative words into more positive phrases; for example, in place of "shooting pain," say "tingling and sparks."
- Describe the sights and sounds around the office.
- Make noises like a dental drill and have the child do the same.

Having the parent act as a fear-free role model for children is often an effective way to help youngsters deal with these anxieties. In one report a four-year-old child was successfully treated by this method (Klesges and Malott 1984). Apparently she had once been frightened by a dentist who had actually slapped her in an attempt to control her during treatment. The trauma was complicated by the fact that the child's mother herself was frightened by dentists. During several "modeling" sessions with a therapist, the mother was asked to demonstrate to the child her lack of anxiety by pretending that she was calm and not afraid. This type of treatment should always be done in careful sequence. In this case, the therapist relied only upon conversation about dentistry for the initial sessions. Then a videotape of a dental visit was shown to both mother and child, and a children's dental game was then played between the therapist and the young girl. Only positive statements were used during each session. Next, there was a tour of a dentist's office, followed by a one-minute checkup. The mother, while role-modeling, pretended to be afraid to get into the dental chair, then sat down, and later said, "It wasn't so bad." At the next session, the child allowed her teeth to be cleaned and X-rayed while sitting on her mother's lap. Finally she allowed full anesthesia and dental repairs to be performed without showing undue anxiety.

Follow-up tests confirmed a dramatic decrease in anxiety in both the mother and child, a classic example of the benefits of behavioral therapy. Combined with supplements for additional backup, such therapy can be rapidly successful. The combination of dental exposure and modeling has been highly effective in treating dental phobias in both adults and children. It's important to remember that with youngsters parental statements, attitudes, and behavior definitely set the tone. If these factors are not altered and continue to be presented negatively to the child, they will contribute greatly to ongoing childhood fears.

Suggested Nutritional Supplements That Can Be Used for Children Over Five with Dentist's Approval

1. Liquid calcium, 300 mg
2. Liquid choline, ½ teaspoon

3. Tryptophan, one 500 mg tablet crushed and put in juice
4. Thiamine, one 25 mg tablet crushed and put in juice

Use the above four items one hour before the dental treatment.
Other items that might help:
Sleepy Time tea, 1 cup
Passion Flower, 1 tablet or capsule
Niacinamide-B$_6$ (by Standard Process Labs), 1 capsule
Rescue, 10 ml. bottle, several drops under tongue when anxious
2 chewable baby aspirins

13

How to Conquer Medical Fears: Fear of Hospitals, Anesthesia, Blood Transfusions, Senility

SCARED OF THE DOCTOR?

Some people show up for a doctor's appointment (after a few post-ponements) in a state of mild terror. Most of the time their fears revolve around the possibility of pain, or discomfort, but the patients also tremble at the thought of the doctor's finding something wrong. Rational thinking and reassurances don't alleviate much of the anxiety, for with medical phobias, the sight of a white coat sends logic flying out the window.

Fear of breast cancer is probably one of the most common reasons why women *do not* see their doctors often enough. They don't want to deal with a confirmation of their worst fears. For some, this anxiety becomes a fatal mistake.

Small children are notoriously fearful of doctors, often crying the minute they walk through the door and, even when calmed, re-maining overly alert for any suspicious moves by the medical staff or their parents. Usually, such fears are initiated by a prior painful experience at a tender age.

If you suspect you have fears related to your health, take this easy test.

MEDICAL FEAR TEST

	YES	NO

Do you have a fear of:

1. Open wounds?
2. Dead people?
3. Insane people?
4. Dentists?
5. People with deformities?
6. Seeing other people injected?
7. Seeing a person being bullied?
8. Dead animals?
9. Physical confrontation?
10. Sick people?
11. Witnessing surgery?
12. Blood?
13. Expecting surgery?
14. Medical odors?
15. Cemeteries?
16. Doctors?
17. Irregular heartbeats?
18. Weapons?
19. Tough-looking people?
20. Seeing people injured?

Scoring the Test

If you scored 50 percent, you probably have the beginnings of a phobia about health care; if your score reached 60 percent or more, you are definitely a medical phobic.

FEAR OF NEEDLES

This is probably one of the most common of all fears, especially among the young. It has been estimated that fourteen out of every 100 people under twenty years old have an abnormal fear of needles or paraphernalia related to injections, but most seem to outgrow it with time. In adults, about five out of every 100 people are still significantly fearful of needles and blood (Costello 1982). Doctors call this fear "blood-injury-illness phobia."

Many people with a fear of needles report feeling faint when confronted with anxiety-producing conditions, much the same as those who have panic attacks; but actual episodes of fainting are limited only to blood-and-injury-phobic patients. In a group of 300 patients, only patients with medical phobias actually fainted, which clearly differentiates them from panic patients (Thyer and Curtis 1983). Both the medical-phobic patients and the panic patients complained of feeling faint to the point where they were about to pass out, but only the needle-phobic patients actually did lose consciousness.

Panic patients typically have an increased heart and respiration rate during their attacks which preclude them from fainting, while it appears that the medical-phobic patients experience just the opposite. Loss of consciousness in these patients is immediately preceded by a rapid decrease in pulse rate, some irregular heartbeats, then a drop in blood pressure.

The pattern turns out to be a little more complicated than one might think at first glance. The reason for the failing heart is due to a rebounding from strong adrenal arousal. When the fearful situation first presents itself, there is an initial burst of anxiety and adrenal arousal. The adrenal gland floods the body with adrenaline, which increases heart rate and blood pressure just as it does in the panic patient. But in the needle-phobic, instead of the gradual decline in excitement and return to normal, there is a quick drop in heart rate and blood pressure, to the point where the patients actually faint.

Out Like a Light

Why does blood pressure drop so rapidly in this group? It is thought that these individuals have an overly strong parasympathetic nervous system. In other words, the excitement, fight-or-flight side of our nervous system, which responds to the sight of a needle, is quickly overpowered by our vegetative (parasympathetic) nervous system, which is trying to calm our excitement. In normal people, this calming side is supposed to bring our nervous system very slowly back down to normal. In the needle-phobic, however, the parasympathetic or calming side of the nervous system overreacts and knocks the excitement side of our nervous system out completely. It doesn't just lower the blood pressure, it knocks it through to the floor. With no blood pressure, there is no oxygen to the brain, and whoosh—out like a light goes the patient.

There are many other types of patients who faint easily and may also have similar mechanisms. Soldiers who stand at attention too long on the parade grounds sometimes faint because their blood has pooled in the lower part of their body, and their heart can no longer pump it into the brain. The causes are not identical to those occurring in needle-phobics, but the same treatment works for both. Those who faint because of heat or claustrophobia fall into roughly the same category and will also respond to the following treatments, as will patients who faint from pain or in response to emotional shock.

There is another possible reason why all of these people faint so easily. It may be due to a deficiency of a neurohormone that helps maintain blood vessel strength. Noradrenaline is a neurohormone that helps maintain blood pressure. When its precursor, tyrosine, is insufficient, the body will be vulnerable to blood pressure instability.

TREATMENT FOR THOSE WHO FAINT EASILY

Nutritional Approach

1. Calcium lactate, 500 mg tablets, 3 or 4 one hour before visiting doctor's office

2. Magnesium, one 100 mg tablet, one hour before visiting doctor's office

The following supplements will be of additional help if your doctor does not object to their use:

3. Tyrosine, one 500 mg tablet 3 times the day before the doctor's visit, and two an hour before the appointment

4. Phenylalanine, 500 mg tablet, a half tablet 3 times a day, and one tablet an hour before seeing the doctor

5. A useful medication is propranolol, a prescription drug that has been used successfully in a number of related cases. Your doctor can tell you how best to use it.

EMERGENCY COPING DEVICES

- For immediate relief, place your head between your knees first and then lie down.
- One of the most useful treatments is to create a feeling of anger when in the presence of a frightening object, for one strong emotion will overcome another. Identify an appropriate fantasy that makes you as angry as possible.

HOME TREATMENTS—EXERCISE NO. 1

Bring to mind the feared object, then quickly replace it with your anger fantasy. Repeat this over and over until the fear does not return.

EXERCISE NO. 2

Another way to dissipate fear is to become gradually desensitized.

1. A plastic syringe and a needle are shown to the patient by the doctor or nurse.

2. The patient is told to take the syringe and needle home and get acquainted with them. A friend or relative can help out if you wish.

3. The patient applies the needle lightly and painlessly to an area of the arm. Go at your own pace—don't rush.

4. When you feel brave enough, return to the doctor's office for a superficial injection in the arm with a short, thin needle. An insulin needle is very good for this, and a sympathetic nurse in the doctor's office can assist you.

5. A small amount of xylocaine (a local anesthetic) is injected under the skin of the arm by the physician. Most doctors are usually glad to cooperate when they understand the problem. This is a gradual approach, and when done with the help of the nutritional supplements and/or medications, success is ensured.

FEAR OF ILLNESS

Thanatophobia, fear of death; nosophobia, fear of having a fatal illness; monophobia, fear of one thing; lysophobia, fear of losing one's mind. These strange names and many others are applied to those who fear a particular aspect of illness. One patient of mine gradually developed such a fear after the following traumatic incident.

"I was standing outside the YMCA talking to friends when one person suddenly looked up, and his face registered horror as he shouted, 'That man is going to jump!' I looked up just in time to glimpse someone leaping off an eighteen-story building. He fell screaming to his death; at the base of the building he landed on a wall, striking it exactly halfway across his body at the midsection. He was torn half in two and his guts spilled out onto the street. I went limp. I felt like I was going to faint. I wanted to sit down, I wanted to throw up. I felt like passing out, but most of all, I didn't want to be there."

An illness phobia is the fear of a specific illness experienced by a healthy individual. It is not the same thing as hypochondriasis, which is a general anxiety over one's health. In such cases, the complaints are multiple and endless and are seldom focused on one disorder. There is another type of disorder that may also be mistaken for an illness phobia, and that is a paranoid delusion. An example would be a fear of being poisoned, with the dastardly deed always just about to take place.

An illness phobia usually involves fear of a current serious illness such as venereal disease, cancer, heart disease, or AIDS—whatever disease happens to be in the limelight. Medical students are famous for worrying about each disease they are studying. Cancerophobic patients usually avoid any place where they think a cancer patient may have been (buses or other public transportation, public toilets, telephones, stores, doctors' offices). If they hear that someone has cancer in a particular location of the body, they imagine they have it in the same region. No physical examinations or lab tests will relieve their minds. Medication helps calm their anxious state, but they are just as fearful when the medication wears off and often become very depressed and morbid. This phobia can become such an obsession that its victims think of nothing else. A classic example is Howard Hughes, who was obsessed with avoiding germs.

Those Are My Symptoms

A phobic patient fears reaching a certain age if family members have died of a particular disease at that age. If there is any disease present, no matter how innocuous, these individuals become convinced it is the beginning of the end. Every deviation from normal has them running to the doctors. There is the story about the singer Al Jolson, who was a notorious hypochondriac. Once at a dinner party, a doctor friend, for amusement, teased him by saying there was a new disease around in which the classic symptoms were a total absence of pain or malaise. These people had absolutely no idea they might be ill. Al Jolson turned white and dropped his fork. "My God," he said, "those are my symptoms exactly!"

Sometimes morbid fears appear after the death of someone close. One young lady developed a fear of bone cancer after her best friend had an amputation to combat the disease. Unfortunately, the surgery did not halt her friend's cancer, and she finally succumbed. The cancer-phobic friend then began regular visits of her own to the doctor. Any leg cramp or charley horse would set her shaking and trembling. While pregnant, she developed frequent leg cramps and was convinced she had cancer brought on by her vulnerable condition. She eventually sought psychiatric help; but many do not, for they refuse to believe that their problems are psychological.

It may seem odd that even such a simple and painless procedure as having one's blood pressure taken can cause apprehension in severely sensitive persons. These patients all seem to be overly attentive to bodily sensations. Like those who have a fear of flying and are supersensitive to every noise or movement of the plane, their obsessive vigilance makes them constantly question the slightest irregularity. They seem unwilling or unable to accept any sensation as par for the course. To them, everything means SOMETHING, in capital letters, with an outcome ranging from grim to disastrous.

Medical-illness phobias seem to fall into that gray area between phobia and anxiety and obsessive-compulsive problems. It's like the old Ink Blot test where, if you look at the drawing one way, you see a rabbit, and if you look at it another way, you see an old lady. Since obsessive-compulsive people seem to suffer from underlying depression, antidepressants or nutritional supplements that reverse depression are often useful. The most difficult part, of course, is getting these people to view their problem as a mental rather than a physical one.

Help for Medical-Illness Phobics

Admit to yourself what is happening. Recognize and accept your fears and take responsibility for them. An illness-phobic who worries about dozens of incidents each week and hundreds if not thousands each year is *not normal*. Admit the problem and deal with it.

Seek out accurate information about any illness that you fear, but try to develop objectivity. You must not dwell on the negative aspects and grim outcomes that can occur, but rather you must spend more time understanding the realities of the disease. For example, if you suspect you have valley fever, but you live at the beach, then use your intelligence and realize that if you truly had the disease, you'd probably make the *Guinness Book of World Records*. Try to change your way of thinking from possibilities to probabilities. If you're feeling under the weather, it's *possible* that you're coming down with bubonic plague, but *probable* that at worst you've got a case of the flu. Your doctor certainly can give you guidance, but so can other therapists and support groups, so take advantage of their help.

When thoughts occur to you, such as, "I wonder if that dark spot on my cheek is cancer," first accept the fact that you had the thought, then be critical of it. Don't just breeze on into "Why is it happening to me?" Resist the temptation to fantasize about all the possible dire consequences, from losing part of your face to a horrific death. Instead, say to yourself, "Why should I have a cancer there?" There's no mole on that spot, and you haven't been irritating it. There is no reason for it to be malignant. Age spots and skin blemishes occur on people's bodies constantly throughout their lives; the chances are very slim that such a blemish is going to do you in. Tell yourself, "I'll just keep an eye on it, but I won't sweat bullets over it."

Another way you can deal with negative thoughts is to clench your fist tightly for three minutes and think only of the fist, nothing else. Watch your knuckles whiten up. Feel the tension and try to bring more strength into your hand. If one hand tires out before the three minutes are up, then start clenching the other hand and do the same thing. Pay attention to what's happening. Just to make sure you use this technique properly, practice it deliberately for three minutes, four times a day.

Refer to the techniques for thought stopping on p. 240. This is an excellent coping device to reduce the amount of attention you place on your health.

Your goal should be to have fewer and fewer thoughts about your health. You could try, for example, to reduce such worries to only about 10 percent of what they now are. One excellent method for accomplishing this is Paradoxical Intention. You'll find instructions for this technique on p. 81.

If you feel your fears are not complex, you could try this simple desensitization routine. It uses the example of having your blood pressure taken, but you can easily substitute any other procedure that troubles you.

Desensitization Schedule

1. Look at a card with the words "blood pressure" written on it until you feel you have no anxiety.

2. Look at a card with BLOOD PRESSURE written on it in very large letters until you feel comfortable.

3. Have someone place a blood pressure cuff three feet from you and leave it there until your fears subside. It's important to keep staring at it. Examine it in detail.

4. Now watch as your helper handles it, keeping it at the same safe distance.

5. Watch your helper place the cuff on another person and test his blood pressure. Repeat this until you feel comfortable.

6. Take the cuff in your hands, then hand it back. Repeat this until you're not afraid.

7. Take the cuff and keep it a minute, then hand it back. Repeat until comfortable.

8. Have your helper place it on your arm, then remove it. Repeat this until comfortable.

9. Finally, have your friend take your blood pressure. Repeat this procedure until it becomes "old hat."

Nutritional Help

Tyrosine, one 500 mg tablet, 3 times a day
Phenylalanine, one 500 mg tablet, 3 times a day
Tryptophan, one 500 mg tablet. May be increased to two tablets, 3 times a day and at bedtime, if it doesn't cause drowsiness.
Niacinamide, 500 mg 3 times a day
B_6, 50 mg 3 times a day
Additional Help
Thiamine, 200 mg 3 times a day
Choline, 500 mg 3 times a day
Calcium lactate, 500 mg 3 times a day and at bedtime

FEAR OF BLUSHING, VOMITING, OR SWEATING

Most people whose fears fall into this category have only one of those anxieties to deal with, but this can become a troublesome problem. Typically fears come on gradually, but they also result from a trauma.

Erythrophobia is the scientific name for fear of blushing. Hyperhidrosis is the term used for excessive perspiration; those with it fear they will profusely sweat in the presence of others. Both disorders are a conditioned automatic reflex. That means they occur automatically and without warning in social situations, are not controllable, and are severe enough to be noticeable to others. The attention one receives creates additional nervousness, and consequently more sweating or blushing. Both of these syndromes are frequently associated with shyness and social phobias.

Psychogenic vomiting is a recognized clinical syndrome, and it occurs in the absence of any known organic pathology. This is not the self-induced vomiting of bulimia patients, but rather the involuntary vomiting in front of others that causes embarrassment. In afflicted persons, retching can be triggered automatically if someone nearby starts to gag or vomit, or it may happen for practically no reason at all. Since this behavior can be extremely offensive to others, these individuals are constantly on guard to avoid any possible trigger. Their only protection is constant vigilance.

Treatment Suggestions

Probably the most effective treatment to date for these phobias is Paradoxical Intention. For thirty days straight, stand in front of a mirror once or twice daily for ten minutes and actively try to create your symptoms. If blushing is the problem, try to make yourself blush; if excessive sweating is the problem, attempt to sweat; and try to vomit if vomiting is your vulnerability. But in this latter category, don't use any physical means to induce vomiting; rely only on psychological manipulations. Also, in the case of vomiting, it's important that you discover where the relevant tensions originate in your body. Then, your object is to create tensions deliberately in these areas. If you're not sure exactly how to do this after reading about Paradoxical Intention on p. 81, then seek professional coaching on the subject.

When you're in a social situation, stop trying to fight your symptoms, and stop avoiding situations that cause the blushing, sweating, or vomiting. At the critical moment, use the Paradoxical Intention technique you have been practicing at home in front of the mirror.

NUTRITION

One hour prior to a social engagement, take the following supplements:

1. Thiamine, 500 mg
2. Niacinamide, 500 mg
3. Aspirin, three grains
4. Calcium lactate, 2,000 mg
5. Choline, 500 mg
6. B$_6$, 50 mg
7. Mintran, 3 tablets

If you have fear of vomiting, you could try

- Ginger root: shave ½ ounce and eat slowly
- Medications prescribed by your physician
- Propranolol, which can be used with or without nutritional supplements. Your doctor will have to prescribe it.

HYPERVENTILATION SYNDROME

In a crowded elevator, a woman suddenly begins to get restless and develops a strange look on her face. She starts to breathe heavily and with difficulty. Others on the elevator become alarmed. The woman shouts that she can't breathe. Finally, the doors to the elevator open and Good Samaritans assist the panicky woman to a chair in the lobby, while someone else calls the paramedics.

Is the woman having a heart attack? A stroke? Fortunately, one onlooker pulls a paper bag out of her purse and hands it to the desperate woman who is gasping for air. She is told to close the bag over her mouth and nose and slowly breathe in and out. Before the paramedics arrive, the panicky woman is well again and ready to go on her way. What she has recovered from is an attack of hyperventilation.

Reports of "overbreathing" go back as far as the sixteenth century, and today it affects about 6 to 11 percent of all patients seen in general practice. The triggers are usually a response to anxiety and/ or improper breathing. The symptoms generally include chest pains, breathlessness, tingling in the hands and around the mouth, disturbed consciousness, feelings of faintness, and suffocating panic. The attacks can come when a person is at rest, or they can sometimes be triggered by a particular incident, such as a crowded elevator, awakening, or falling asleep.

Causes of Hyperventilation

1. *Organic*
   Drug intoxication   Alcohol withdrawal
   Aspirin overdose   Sugar withdrawal

2. *Physiological*
   Exercise   Heat
   Altitude

3. *Emotional*
   Closed places   Guilt
   Pain   Sorrow
   Unpleasant thoughts   Anxiety
   Anger and resentment

4. *Habit*
   Respiratory irregularity   Sighing
   Sub-breathing   Overbreathing

Treatment for Hyperventilation

During the attack, a simple brown bag is a lifesaver, so keep one on your person at all times.

Be aware of the triggers I have listed above and avoid them when necessary. For example, sugar, colas, cigarettes, alcohol, and recreational drugs can all trigger fear attacks, as can food allergies.

Reread Chapter 3 on triggers, and try to relate them to yourself. Avoid or neutralize those which you feel affect you.

MEDITATION

If you tend to be an on-edge, Type-A personality, try to work toward developing a more tranquil outlook. Meditation is probably the best-known method of self-regulation and self-control. It works by inducing an altered state of consciousness as well as a state of relaxation. It is a wakeful, hypometabolic physiological state. The transcendental meditation (TM) technique is probably the most widely known. Mahar Ihi Mahesh Yogi teaches another technique that is practiced by over a million people each day.

Meditation has proved useful in cases of claustrophobia, pain control, and various kinds of phobias, and may be used along with other procedures. It could be considered a type of global desensitization, where one views all events in a relaxed state of mind. On the other hand, the benefits may result from simply taking time out from daily affairs to remove general stress, thus promoting conditions for the body's automatic relaxation response to occur.

Major requirements:

- Quiet environment
- Decreased muscle tone
- A mental device to help shift the mind away from ordinary, rational thought processes
- A passive attitude toward meditation; don't worry about how well you are performing the technique, just disregard any distracting thoughts.

There are a number of paperback books that teach this method, and tapes are also available. Your local bookstore should be able to help. There are also classes available in most major cities, and you'll find them advertised in the paper or listed in the yellow pages of your telephone directory. Transcendental meditation has been well tested, so you should have little concern about its effectiveness, assuming it appeals to you. If it doesn't happen to be your cup of tea, try listening to a daily tape.

PLEASURE READING

Believe it or not, some researchers have found regularly scheduled pleasure reading to be as effective as meditation in relieving anxiety. For this to work, sit quietly without engaging in any specific mental activity except the creation of positive daydreams. Just read at your normal pace, and really get into it with your imagination.

This is the way it works:

- It causes the relaxation response to occur.
- It causes you to disengage yourself from the world.
- It's pleasurable.
- It reestablishes a sense of control.

Like other forms of therapy, pleasure reading works only when you do it regularly, so be sure you set aside some time for yourself each day or at least every other day.

PARADOXICAL INTENTION

This has been a very successful method in the treatment of all forms of anxiety, so review Chapter 4 on general treatment, and apply this coping technique whenever you experience the first signs of anxiety.

BREATHING EXERCISES

Review the breathing exercises in Chapter 4, and practice them daily in order to regain control of your breathing. These techniques, plus learning how to breathe using different muscles, will make you much less susceptible to hyperventilation. Pharmacies now carry a small plastic device that asthmatics use to practice breathing, and it's quite useful in building up control to prevent hyperventilation.

NUTRITIONAL SUPPLEMENTS

1. One aspirin, prior to entering any area or situation that might trigger an attack
2. Thiamine, 200 mg, 3 times a day
3. Calcium lactate, 500 mg, 3 times a day and at bedtime
4. Choline, 1,000 mg, 3 times a day and at bedtime

5. Niacinamide, two tablets (B_6), by Standard Process Labs, 3 times a day and at bedtime
6. Tryptophan, 500 mg, 3 times a day

Use all of these supplements one hour before foreseeable exposure to any known trigger.

14

How to Conquer Nightmares, Night Terrors, Daymares

Although studies indicate that night terrors are a severe disorder, rarely do sufferers seek help. Most doctors only hear about disturbing dreams incidentally during routine exams. According to research, nightmares, night terrors, and "day" mares are caused by separate mechanisms, but in my clinical experience, proper nutritional techniques can control all of them quite well.

NIGHTMARES

First, let's identify each entity. A nightmare is usually a complete dream that is frightening throughout or becomes frightening enough at the end to cause the individual to awaken in a terrified state. Nightmares most often involve some sort of chase, with the dreamer trying to avoid violence or death. Seldom does the dream portray actual dangers, past or present. The most prominent symptom is the pervasive feeling of helplessness that accompanies such panic. The nightmare usually occurs near the end of the sleep period, and even though the person goes back to sleep, he will probably remember the dream the following morning.

265

NIGHT TERRORS

In contrast, those suffering night terrors do not remember the experience. Those who undergo night terrors usually signal their ordeal with a terrorized scream but do not awaken at that point. The few who remember anything the following day merely recall sensations of suffocation or pressure on the chest. Someone who tries to awaken them will find it extremely difficult because night terror patients are groggy and hard to bring around. Night terrors usually occur early in the night, often not long after the person has fallen asleep. As he or she screams and possibly sits up, there are major changes in physiology. The heart races and breathing rate doubles.

Night terrors are not dreams; they are a startling sensation. Body movements accompanying the scream can include sleepwalking. Night terrors have been created in susceptible children simply by pulling them upright while asleep. They have also been created in posttraumatic nightmare patients in the same manner. Because it's possible to induce a startled reaction in these individuals, there is considered to be a relationship between the two disorders. Night terror patients, not remembering their nocturnal experiences, usually discover their problem only when another person tells them about it, or if they sleepwalk and awaken in an unfamiliar location. Posttraumatic nightmare patients, however, usually do recall their dreams. Some patients suffer both phenomena, nightmares and night terrors. I will discuss sleepwalking as it relates to night terrors a little later.

Posttraumatic Nightmare

Posttraumatic nightmares occur, supposedly, as a consequence of some frightening event, such as a war experience or a rape or attack. This type of bad dream seems to be a cross between a nightmare and a night terror, but biochemically, it's closer to night terror. The patient reexperiences the terrible event as a dream, which he can later remember, but he may also sit up with a scream or walk in his sleep. Posttraumatic nightmares are rather common and can occur at any age.

A Common Problem

It's impossible to say how many people suffer from nightmares or night terrors, but it's safe to say that they number in the millions. While occasional nightmares are probably universal, those who suffer them frequently represent about 5 to 10 percent of the population.

Nightmares occur frequently in children aged three to six, but they have been noted in those even younger. It's thought that as many men as women suffer from this disorder; but since fewer men seek help, it's more often thought of as a "woman's disease." In my experience, because of the possible destabilizing effect of the menstrual cycle, women are probably a bit more vulnerable than men. Although the tendency to nightmares and night terrors seems to wane with age, older individuals are not immune.

Sleepwalking

Although nightmares are not dangerous, sleepwalking can result in injury or even death. A young man once fell asleep and awakened several hours later, standing in front of his front door bleeding from a head injury (Rouch and Stern 1986). Apparently he had been walking in his sleep and had fallen twenty feet from his second-story porch into some bushes below. Another patient, the same researchers report, wakened to find blood spurting from his wrist—he was stuck halfway through a broken, glass sliding door!

Complex behavior in addition to simple sleepwalking can also occur during these episodes. A case in point is that of a young man who was given to striking out at people or smashing furniture during violent episodes while sleepwalking. In these instances, he was not only a threat to himself, but a danger to others (Hartman 1983). His wife had been brutally battered during several nocturnal attacks, and it was feared he might seriously injure their infant child. One of the most serious cases described in the same report involved a fifty-year-old man, who, feeling tired, pulled his car into a highway rest area for a brief nap. An hour later, he sat up and started his car, but apparently he was not awake at the time. He drove onto the highway in the wrong direction into oncoming traffic. Drivers swerved all over the road to avoid a collision, and horns blared as other motorists tried to alert him. But the man continued driving, staring straight ahead in a fixed, zombielike manner. Eventually he crashed head-on into a car, killing its three occupants.

The Alcohol Connection

There are some known triggers that can precipitate nightmares and night terrors. Most noticeable in this group is alcohol, and I will address this important subject again later in the chapter. The man who fell off his porch was a heavy beer drinker. The man who cut his wrist walking through a glass door drank excessively on weekends. It was not noted whether the third man drank, but in the fourth and most serious case, the man was a moderate social drinker, who occasionally indulged more heavily. On the day of the accident, he had consumed five or six cocktails prior to the drive.

Other "Triggers" to Nightmares

Nightmares may occur during fever or illnesses, both physical and mental; encephalitis is associated with nightmares, as is the onset of psychosis. It has been found that nightmares are associated more frequently with psychoses, particularly schizophrenia, than with neuroses. I have seen many cases of nightmares associated with hormone imbalance, such as premenstrual syndrome, and also with increased anxiety states, such as panic attacks and agoraphobia. Depression is another condition which can bring on nightmares in susceptible individuals.

Among the drugs that can trigger nightmares, the most potent is L-dopa, an amino-acid medication which has been used to treat Parkinson's disease. Beta-blockers, such as propranolol, used to correct heart pathology and treat high blood pressure also cause nightmares. Street drugs are especially risky for certain individuals. Withdrawal from both street drugs and prescription medications including tranquilizers can also result in violent dreams.

Stress may also trigger nightmares, especially in the instance of location changes, job changes, sleep deprivation, or the loss of someone close. The most important dynamic of the stressful situation that often produces nightmares is the feeling of helplessness. If the attitude and disposition of the individual is basically negative, it adds to the potential problem. Individuals who see only the grim side of life or who dwell on thoughts of death or calamity are naturally going to be more inclined to have nightmares.

Personalities of Nightmare Patients

The basic characteristics of those with night terrors have not been defined, but those experiencing frequent nightmares are often sensitive and creative people inclined toward moodiness and depression. Most are ambitious, but also rebellious and independent. Many are so biochemically sensitive that they do not fare well with drugs, either prescription or recreational. For these individuals, even small quantities of an offending substance can produce adverse effects.

But in general, it can be said that the vast majority of those who suffer from sleep afflictions are people who show very few psychological abnormalities. Some researchers have tried to find definitive psychological patterns, but without success. People with these sleep difficulties often have associated sleep problems, such as bedwetting, nocturnal grinding of jaws (bruxism), and insomnia. Sleep apnea and/or snoring have not been closely associated with these disorders, but I have seen patients in whom they have occurred simultaneously.

DAYMARES

Daymares are terrifying daydreams that are real enough to cause auto accidents if they occur while a person is driving. One of my patients, who experiences night terrors, nightmares, and daymares, becomes very vulnerable when she is fatigued. On a particularly difficult day, following a week of nonstop work and little sleep, she was driving down a freeway and was horrified to find herself about to run down a group of people who were walking directly in front of her. She jammed on the brakes and careened across the freeway, causing cars to scatter in all directions. Fortunately, it was not a busy time of day, and all of the frightened drivers managed to miss one another. When she pulled to the side of the road to stop and to look back at the crowd she had narrowly missed, she found that they did not exist! At the moment she saw them, however, they appeared to be totally real.

Daymares are most often dreams of disaster and frequently accompany feelings of desertion, fear of failure, or impending doom. Panic occurs as palms sweat, breathing rate increases, and muscles tense. Because daymares are dreamlike, they can be linked to nightmares, and categorized in the same group of disorders.

THE MECHANISM OF NORMAL SLEEP

Nightmares occur during the portion of the sleep cycle which produces rapid eye movements (REM). Most people go through four or five 90-minute cycles of sleep each night. Like a roller coaster, they go into a deep sleep, then rise to a near wakefulness, then drop down again to deep sleep, and so on. In the REM phase, the sleep is at the top of the roller coaster ride—close to wakefulness—so physiological changes occur. In addition to rapid eye movements, the pulse increases, and breathing speeds up. Blood pressure may rise and muscle tone decreases. At this point, it may be difficult to rouse the sleeper.

Neurotransmitters—Very Important for Normal Sleep or Nightmares

We have discussed amino acids and neurotransmitters previously (see Chapter 4), so you should remember that neurotransmitters are chemical messengers that allow one nerve to activate another. There are four neurotransmitters that relate to both sleep and nightmares: dopamine, acetylcholine, noradrenaline, and serotonin. The changing balance of the amounts of these neurotransmitters contributes to normal sleep and normal dreams. Abnormal changes in these balances are suspected by some to be the cause of nightmares. It appears that serotonin and noradrenaline are balanced against the other two neurohormones, acetylcholine and dopamine. During REM sleep, serotonin and noradrenaline are low, while dopamine and acety-choline are higher. When these neurohormones are balanced properly, normal dreams occur.

Dreams Serve a Purpose

No one is certain just why we dream; the process may simply be a by-product of the restorative biochemical functions of sleep. In that case, dreams could serve as a sign of good psychological health, a necessity for the assimilation of life's stresses. The time spent sleeping allows the mind time to sort things out and organize events in a practical and useful way. In this sense, then, dreams are not just helpful, but essential.

But dreams have another function too; they may serve to keep one asleep. Rather than becoming aroused by certain stimuli, a dreamer is distracted by a fantasy which protects and prolongs his retreat from the world. Nightmares are abnormal dreams, so in a sense they are an out-of-balance dream, which may be a reflection of out-of-balance biochemistry.

My Personal Experiences

Like other physicians, I have developed some of my own treatments with my own rationales as to why they work. I cannot always prove why these methods are effective; all I know is that they do the job. Reading over research materials, I found that other physicians have made similar observations, but some have come to different conclusions and have different hypotheses.

Alcohol

The use of alcohol has often been associated with nightmares. I believe it works in two ways. First of all, alcohol is notorious for destroying thiamine. The loss of this vitamin and others causes many of the health problems related to alcoholism. Lonsdale has reported the onset of nightmares when thiamine is depleted. Second, I believe that alcohol also changes the calcium-potassium ratio in the blood, so that a relative potassium deficiency develops. Potassium-deficient people are not only tired, they actually become groggy, and have great difficulty awakening in the morning or from a deep sleep. They are often not fully awake for a full hour after arising. In a sense, these individuals are almost sleepwalking, for it's a consistent finding that sleepwalkers are hard to awaken. The sleepwalker mentioned earlier in this chapter fell twenty feet from a porch and injured his head, then got up and walked all the way to his front door *before* waking up! The similarity between the grogginess caused by potassium deficiency and the grogginess of nightmare victims is too marked to ignore.

Stress seems to be another precipitant of nightmares. The connection between stress and psychological implications has already been illuminated in medical literature. What hasn't been emphasized is that stress depletes and unbalances nutritional balance. Since it is scientifically correct to say that neurohormone balance is pertinent to normal sleep, it also makes sense that the coenzymes to the neurohormones, vitamins and minerals, must also be in proper balance for normal sleep. Included among the substances that destabilize coenzymes are alcohol, stress, and that favorite American staple, caffeine.

Caffeine

Caffeine is anti-thiamine. It destroys vitamins, especially when consumed in large amounts. Caffeine's second effect is to act as a diuretic. Loss of fluid from the body produces a loss of potassium, magnesium, and numerous other nutrients. Although the diuretic effect differs from one person to another, in general it occurs when caffeine intake is high. Excessive use can make one allergic, sometimes causing bladder irritation, relieved only by frequent urination.

The person who just can't seem to get going in the morning without a pot of coffee may be a victim of this vicious cycle. Coffee depletes or unbalances potassium, magnesium, and other nutrients, causing fatigue and grogginess which the victim tries to counteract by drinking still more caffeine or colas. At the same time he may be altering his sleep cycle by changing the neurohormone and coenzyme balances. Excessive use of any substance can upset delicate body chemistry and is not a wise practice.

Foods Do Cause Nightmares

In the part of the book relating to triggers, I discuss food allergies as a trigger to fear-level disturbances. Both clinicians and the lay public have suspected that certain foods may cause nightmares. There have been no in-depth studies on this subject, however, so it's difficult to make precise correlations. Gastrointestinal irritation has been considered the actual exciter, if such is the case. I believe that the nightmares people have after eating certain foods are due more to allergies than from overreactions to the foods themselves. I have seen several cases where elimination of the offending food from the diet seems to reduce the frequency of nightmares.

Drugs and Chemical Nightmares

Reaction to chemicals is another source of biochemical imbalance. Smoke, formaldehydes, phenols, and other chemicals are known to interfere with the functions of the enzyme systems. Since enzymes control biochemical interactions, any blockage can produce symptoms. I have seen no such related cases, but I believe that chemical sensitivity does contribute to nightmares. The closest correlation I've come across is the fact that those who have nightmares are frequently hypersensitive to street drugs (Hartman 1984). Even small amounts of marijuana can cause nightmares in individuals. If oral toxins can produce this type of reaction, then certainly inhaled or contact chemicals can do the same.

Aspirin—The Magic Wand

A dose of 650 mg of aspirin increases sleep time and decreases wakefulness in insomniacs. Aspirin has a mild sedative/hypnotic effect. It appears to improve sleep significantly in the second half of the night as there seems to be a four-hour delay before the hypnotic activity takes place.

Suanzaorentang—The Magic Carpet

Suanzaorentang is an ancient Chinese herbal remedy for insomnia. Taking 1,000 mg thirty minutes before bedtime significantly improved the sleep of sixty patients who all suffered sleep disorders. The bonus of this remedy was that most of the people felt much better the next day. They reported a reduction in palpitations, anxiety, neck stiffness, perspiration, and low back pains, as well as an increased sense of well-being (Chen and Hsieh 1985).

Steps to Control Nightmares

What are the steps one can take to control these sleep problems?

1. Two 500 mg potassium tablets at 4 P.M.
    One 250 mg B_1 tablet at bedtime
    One 1,000 mg choline tablet at bedtime
    One 1,000 mg niacinamide tablet at bedtime

2. Discover any food allergies and eliminate them (see Chapter 3 on triggers).

3. Avoid or use with caution any prescription drug known to induce nightmares, such as reserpine, propranolol (Inderol), L-dopa, and phenothiazine. Request information on any drugs used to treat angina, hypertension, or Parkinsonism. If you are troubled by nightmares, all drugs should be used with caution.

4. Antidepressant and antipsychotic medicines reduce nightmares, but they must be prescribed by a physician and watched carefully for side effects.

5. Some tranquilizers also reduce nightmares, but withdrawal from them can cause rebound nightmares.

6. Emotional ventilation, getting it all out—allowing full expression of feeling—may also be helpful. This can be done alone, or in a therapy setting, either privately or with a group.

7.   Behavioral therapy sometimes has been helpful. (See Resources in Chapter 18.)

8.   Psychotherapy has occasionally proved effective.

9.   Alcohol should be completely avoided in the extreme cases, and moderate drinkers can avoid alcohol's negative effects by using the nutritional formula and doubling the dosage on drinking days.

10.   Caffeine should be reduced or eliminated.

11.   Stress will increase the need for the nutritional formula, and during intense periods, you may need to double or triple the dose.

12.   Do not deprive yourself of sleep. Staying up late for either work or pleasure should be avoided.

13.   Fatigue can induce nightmares, whether it results from an extra workout at the gym or unaccustomed labor, such as cleaning out the garage. When one is especially fatigued, the nutritional formula should be increased, as it should be if your job is physically demanding.

14.   Try adding aspirin, suanzaorentang, or nicotine gum to your nutritional supplements.

15

How to Conquer the Fear of "Creatures"

The fear of spiders, dogs, and other animals is experienced on a mild level by most people. These common fears cannot be called phobias unless they interfere with normal living. At the level they exist in most of us, such anxieties are usually controllable. However, a fear of specific animals or insects is one of the most common problems encountered by psychiatrists. For the most part, individuals with these fears are usually otherwise normal, although agoraphobics are particularly vulnerable to developing these fears along with their other symptoms.

The degree of discomfort caused by such a phobia depends on its intensity and how frequently the person has to face the animal or insect that he fears. Generally, it is more of a nuisance than a disability, and the individual's life is not much affected. However, since these fears cause a person to avoid a particular creature at all costs, it can become quite a handicap to fear dogs in a locale where there is a canine on every corner.

People who fall into this category usually complain of long-standing fears of a certain animal or insect but appear to be free of other symptoms. In other words, they don't fear all animals, only one species, and are usually quite comfortable with most forms of life, be they two-, four-, or eight-legged.

This test can give you a quick idea whether or not you are subject to animal phobia.

ANIMAL PHOBIA

	Mild	Moderate	Severe
1. I don't like worms.	————	————	————
2. I don't like insects.	————	————	————
3. I don't like birds.	————	————	————
4. I don't like cats.	————	————	————
5. I don't like bats.	————	————	————
6. I don't like flying insects.	————	————	————
7. I don't like any kind of snake.	————	————	————
8. I don't like mice.	————	————	————
9. I don't like dogs.	————	————	————

If any answers were in the "severe" column, you are probably phobic. One or two answers in the "moderate" column and you may be suspicious of a developing phobia.

Genetics has been suggested as having a role in these fears, since such individuals often appear to have a certain fear-preparedness or else they seem to be constantly incubating fear. But, on the other hand, it has been found that families of these patients are usually stable and fairly well adjusted. Few of the relatives had any suggestion of phobias.

Most animal-phobic patients are perfectly normal until they encounter the creature that terrifies them. Afterwards, they return to normal, until the next time a mouse or a snake rears its ugly head. There are no distinctions in personality types either. Some reports claim that a fair proportion of those patients were fearful as children, that they cried more than others, were more shy and withdrawn, and more prone to bed-wetting. Follow-up studies, however, do not find these people suffering from inferior schoolwork or from occupational handicaps.

Single phobias can develop in any normal person under the right circumstances. For a good example, reread the sections in Chapter 8 on fear of flying and, especially, on fear of driving. Driving fear, which is a single phobia, occurs in normal people after accidents or near-accidents as a learned reflex, and the same can be true of animal phobias, although they don't always develop after a known trauma.

Most patients acquired their animal phobias during childhood, but the majority could not remember its resulting from any specific event. One report showed that 77 percent of those interviewed could not recall the origin of their phobias and simply recalled having experienced their particular fear for as long as they could remember (McNally and Streketee 1985). In 90 percent of the cases, the levels of the patients' fears had always been at the maximum intensity, while 10 percent professed to have gradually increasing fears. All youngsters experience some fears during normal development; but a few fail to outgrow them, and they remain as a persistent remnant of normal childhood fears.

Phobias can originate at any time in a person's life (except infancy); but they usually show up in early childhood, and the great majority begin before the age of seven. Once firmly established, the intensity of the fear remains fixed and constant for 90 percent of sufferers. This means they are not strong one day and weak the next. The level of fear never varies in intensity.

In some vulnerable individuals, the conditioned responses to phobic stimuli are very persistent. It is true that the human species is biologically prepared to be afraid, and man may well have been programmed to associate fear with potentially dangerous creatures such as snakes and spiders, lions and tigers. However, neutral experiences with these stimuli will normally cause the fears to dissipate. According to the conditioning theory of neuroses, fears are acquired through some fearful association with previously neutral stimuli. Such conditioning has a strong role in survival, and therefore is not without purpose.

While the "inborn ability to learn" may allow conditioned reflexes to overreact and phobias to develop, many believe that direct conditioning of any kind accounts for relatively few phobias. As a matter of fact, some experts believe that many fears are acquired on the basis of information transmitted through observation and instruction. In other words, we learn fear from others. Some researchers believe that negative instructions provided by parents and relatives greatly influence phobic development. Vivid stories meant to entertain a child can set off the process, or fears may be passed on by the parents as a form of vicarious learning.

A radio-show host once asked a psychiatrist why elephants are afraid of mice. The doctor explained that it was probably due to the lack of predictability in the rodent's behavior. Although the answer was given for this specific situation, it applies generally to the fear of all animals. Patients often say that they fear animals because they don't know what they will do, and their spontaneous actions surprise and frighten them. Patients are also often afraid of the physical appearance of a particular creature.

Besides fearing animals' lack of predictability, most patients also worry that they might have a panic attack if they have a sudden, unavoidable encounter with a creature that frightens them. The panic attack, besides being unpleasant in itself, would be a source of embarrassment. Others fear that an animal might actually cause them to have a heart attack, and some believe they might be physically attacked and harmed by the beast.

Such fears cause these people to keep an eye out for the animal wherever they go. Even the slightest hint that it might be present can cause anxiety. This means "animal awareness" is a sign of a high fear level. Besides waking fears, some people experience recurring nightmares. Such persons dream that they are bound in some way and cannot escape contact with a dreaded animal. A few patients dwell on their phobias and work themselves into a terrible state of mind. Not being able to shake their compulsive thoughts, they fall into depression.

Birds

When asked to describe the most dangerous bird one might possibly encounter, most people would say a fierce bird of prey, like an eagle or a hawk. But oddly enough, the most widely feared bird of all is the pigeon. Not because there's a certain "risk" involved in walking underneath them, but because many people have been conditioned to fear them.

One patient said, "I hate pigeons. I never leave the house without looking outside to see if there are any around. Then I rush to the car. At home I keep all the windows and doors tightly shut even on the hottest days. I think it might have started when I was a kid. I was going out with some other boys to see a friend. I guess his father didn't like birds, because he set up wire traps—big square cages of wire so that he could catch a hundred birds at a time. As we arrived at my friend's house, he asked us if we wanted to watch something funny. We said yes. His father then picked up one of the cages containing dozens of pigeons and plunged it into a barrel of water. The loud chirps stopped as the cage sank below the water. I was horrified, and my stomach turned flips. I felt weak, and then I dreamed about it all that night and thought about it for days. I guess it was then I first started to be bothered by birds. Maybe I thought they would get back at me. I don't know."

From another patient came this story: "I'm a chicken about chickens. I know they won't hurt me, but I'm afraid of them anyway. When I was a kid, I went to visit my uncle on the farm. My aunt asked me to go to the henhouse and get some eggs. I had seen how she did it, by gently lifting up the hen, so I thought I could do it too. As I entered and closed the gate to the yard, I heard a noise behind me. It was a rooster. It was big and mean and chased me around the yard. My uncle came to watch but wouldn't help. He only laughed. Finally, after what seemed an eternity, he came into the yard and chased away the rooster. My relief didn't last long. He said he came to get dinner; he picked up a chicken and twisted its head off and threw it on the ground. The body kept flopping around spewing blood everywhere. Those few minutes seemed like hours. If I hadn't had the second shock, I probably would have gotten over the rooster attack. Now I keep a sharp eye out for chickens. I won't eat them and I don't like to see pictures of them."

Snakes

In the Bible and mythology snakes have been linked to evil. It's even possible that fear of these sometimes dangerous reptiles is innate. Freud, on the other hand, considered them to be a phallic symbol. To Freud, dreams about them indicated either a fear of intercourse, fear of rape, or a preoccupation with sex.

Although the fear of snakes is not unusual, an analysis of over 100 people who expressed a fear of snakes showed that most phobics had little personal experience with them (Murray and Foote 1979). In fact, the more firsthand experience people actually have with snakes, the braver they become.

There are a lot of things that bother people about snakes because they seem to have very few redeeming qualities—they certainly aren't cuddly! People fear they will be bitten, poisoned, or suffocated, which is not totally unrealistic. And in the instance of harmless snakes, people don't like their appearance, their ability to move silently and stealthily, and their sudden movements. In a small minority of people, there is a fear that a snake might enter a body opening.

Dogs

Ask any postman about dogs, then stand back. Even a small dog can look menacing when he's aroused. One dog phobic says, "When I was little, a friend brought over her big dog, who jumped on me suddenly and knocked me down on the floor. I got so scared and cried so hard they had to take him away. The next thing I remember is thinking how dogs always stared at me. I knew they knew how scared I was; I could see it in their eyes. I became afraid that any dog would bite me. My mother had to take me to school and pick me up. I always had to have someone to go places with, and I hated to even be outdoors. I couldn't get dogs out of my mind. I was always afraid I would encounter one unexpectedly."

We could go on and on to describe the many other animals and insects that patients fear, but after a while, the details begin to sound the same. Any experience during a period of vulnerability can create a fear of a particular animal, and once that happens, a person is stuck with the fear unless he decides to take some action. Before we go on, let's find out how scary a particular creature is to you.

DEGREES OF FEARS OF ANIMALS

Take the test below both before and after you have treated yourself. This comparison will give you some idea of your progress. Think of the animal or insect you fear, then ask yourself which of the following statements describes your reactions best.

1. This does not upset me in any way.
2. I'm a little upset but not much.
3. I'm uneasy about this.
4. I'm especially uneasy about this.
5. I'm frightened about this.
6. I'm very frightened by this.
7. It's too scary to think about.
8. I'm terrified.

Mark down your answer for comparison after you have completed the treatment program.

THE LOGICAL APPROACH

Fill out this questionnaire regarding the feared creature slowly, *thinking each answer through* carefully.

1. List five of your first memories regarding the animal. _____

_____

2. List any fearful dreams. _____

_____

_____

3. Take five minutes and think about all of your actual experiences with the creature, then list the place, time, and a six-word description of what happened (i.e., I ran away, or I fainted). ____

_____

4. What bothers you the most about this animal? List all of his characteristics. _____

_____

_____

5. What actual beliefs do you hold about the animal? (I believe they are all dangerous; I believe they cannot be controlled, etc.) Make one single statement about your attitude. _____

Now go to the local library or bookstore and get a reliable book on snakes (or the particular creature you fear); for example, *Snakes of the World: Their Ways and Means of Living*, by Hampton W. Parker (New York: Dover, 1971), is a particularly informative book. If possible, choose one without a lot of pictures. Read the book and think about your previous conceptions. Reread your statements on the questionnaire.

ONE-DAY CURES

The following excercises have been used to cure a phobia in one long session. For mild to moderate phobias, it may work that quickly, but for intense phobias it will probably take longer.

The treatments use snakes as an example, but they work for any animal or insect. Simply insert the name of the animal or creature about which you wish to become desensitized.

An important instruction: *You have to override any discomfort felt while doing the exercise in the interest of gaining new experiences.*

Sustained Respiratory Relief with a Friend's Help

Note: The physical presence of a particular object makes it impossible to exaggerate or be unrealistic about one's feelings toward it.

1. Have a friend obtain a harmless snake from a pet store.

2. Inhale deeply. Take the air in slowly and completely. Close your eyes. Hold your breath as long as you can. Even when you feel you've reached your limit, hold it a moment more. Place your right palm

over your mouth and pinch your nose with your fingers. Both can be done with one hand.

3. Have your friend bring the snake into the room and place it behind you. During the breath-holding, turn around and, when you can no longer hold your breath, open your mouth and your eyes at the same time. This procedure can be repeated two or three times. Take the snake out of the room before each repetition.

4. It is important that you hold your breath for the maximum time possible. (If you are doing it alone, the tendency will be to quit too soon, before reaching a deep enough state of respiratory arrest.) When done correctly, the urgent need to breathe will override all other anxieties.

5. It is also important that you *look* at the snake and say to yourself, or state out loud, every single thing you have ever thought about snakes.
NOTE: *Your eyes must never leave the snake the entire time you are thinking about it.*

6. Stay with this process as long as you can tolerate it, until most of your anxiety is gone.

7. Repeat this exercise as often as possible.

Variation of the Respiratory Relief Exercise

1. Take twenty breaths in a paper bag. The last breath should completely fill your lungs. Then exhale the air and pinch your nose.

2. Advance toward the object or have it brought toward you. *Warning:* Some people can be made more nervous by carbon dioxide. If you find that your nervousness increases as you breathe in the bag, use a different exercise. Most people, however, will find that they become more relaxed.

3. Take ten more breaths in the paper bag, then slowly edge toward the frightening object, while continuing to breathe into the bag and avoiding all eye contact. Look down or sideways.

4. When you reach the twentieth breath in the bag, do the respiratory arrest: Pinch your nose, open your eyes and look right at the object.

5. Then turn away and wait two minutes.

6. Start again. Take ten breaths in the bag, then turn around with your eyes closed and slowly edge forward, taking more breaths.

7. When you reach twenty breaths, turn away from the feared object. Do the respiratory arrest. Turn around and open your eyes just as you are forced to breathe. Study the creature.

Or you can do the opposite: Have your friend slowly bring the feared animal toward you. View it only after you have held your breath for the maximum amount of time.

Fantasy Session with a Friend's Help

1. Take your fear-scale test before and after the session.

2. Have a friend tape four five-to-seven-minute stories about snakes or whatever animal frightens you. The stories should be as realistic and scary as possible.

3. Sit in an armchair, get comfortable, close your eyes, and let your mind stay with the story on the tapes. The more anxiety you expose yourself to, the sooner you'll be in control.

4. Play tapes in this order: 1-2-1-2-1-2-1-2-1-2-3-4-3-4-3-4-3-4. It would be easier if your friend did it for you. The entire exercise will take about two hours.

Exposure to the Feared Animal

After the session, try to expose yourself to the real object—snakes, cats, birds, etc. Have your friend bring the animal into the house, and then gradually closer to you, in slow stages, over a period of thirty minutes to an hour.

1. Bring the animal to the nearest tolerable location. Wait five to ten minutes until the anxiety subsides. Gauge the level of your fear. Do not bring the animal any closer than a "five" on your fear scale.

2. Again, bring the animal to the next closest tolerable location. Wait five to ten minutes until the anxiety subsides.

3. Continue this pattern until the creature is actually touched. Keep it on your lap for half an hour.

If you still have high fear levels or if your panic returns, repeat this approach one or two more times. Studies have shown that most people are able to achieve good control over their anxiety after one to three sessions.

Going Straight to the Worst Fear First

The following exercise is called a flooding technique: confronting your worst fear right from the outset.

1. Allow for a full half-hour.

2. Get into a comfortable chair.

3. Use all of your senses and powers of imagination to produce scenes involving snakes. (Insert the name of the appropriate animal.) As you go through the scenes, make up a hierarchy, pick the scene that bothers you most to start with, then move on to more frightening scenes. Put the scenes on three-by-five-inch cards, then go through the cards in the order you have arranged.

Examples:

- Picture a slimy snake moving across your hands and arms.
- Imagine a snake crawling around on your stomach; it is trapped and biting you mercilessly.
- A giant snake is attacking you.
- A huge snake is wrapped around your neck and is slowly suffocating you.

You must reach the highest anxiety levels possible. If you get too nervous, open your eyes for a moment, then go back to your images.

Mild and moderate cases may require only one treatment, while severe cases may take several sessions. Take the fear-scale test both before and after the treatment.

Treatment Tricks

Tricking people into thinking they have made progress can actually create improvements. One research team gave false heart-rate readings to patients exposed to snakes. This allegedly calm indicator gave the phobics the impression that they were more relaxed than they really were, and from then on, their fears began to decrease. The conclusion was that if a patient *thinks* he is relaxed around a particular animal, his behavior will change accordingly.

Nutritional Supplements

Another type of phobia is called a single phobia, which means the person with the fear is anxiety-free most of the time. Therefore the formula below need only be used under two sets of circumstances: when one is actually going to be in the presence of the feared animal or insect, or during any desensitization exercise used above. In each case, try to take your supplements one hour before the encounter. It might be wise to carry one dose in a plastic bag in case of an emergency, should you have a surprise run-in with your dreaded critter.

1. Thiamine, one 500 mg tablet
2. Calcium lactate, one 500 mg tablet
3. Mintran, three tablets
4. Niacinamide-B_6, 4
5. Choline, two 1,000 mg tablets
6. Aspirin, 5 grains, one tablet
7. Biotin, three 1 mcg tablets

PART

4

FINAL VIEWS ON THE PROBLEMS OF FEARS

16

The Psychology of Fear

Throughout this book, we have not included much discussion of the classical approach to treating anxiety because this method is being used less and less frequently. The behavioral approach, however, is still a viable and commonly used treatment which has withstood the test of time, and I use some of its techniques along with my nutritional approach. I have already discussed therapy in Chapter 4, so I won't repeat it here. What I will try to do is put the various psychological approaches to anxiety into perspective.

THE PSYCHOANALYTICAL APPROACH TO ANXIETY

The media, with their pervasive influence, tend to depict all psychiatric treatment in terms of the ubiquitous "couch." Films frequently portray a patient receiving help while lying prone in his analyst's office. This image, however, is something of a misconception, for those scenes apply only in the practice of psychoanalysis. While conveniently dramatic for Hollywood's purposes, in actuality this archaic therapy is only used by a few therapists. Psychoanalysts, however, are credited with being the first to create a public awareness of phobias.

According to classical psychoanalytical literature, the first step in the development of a phobia is the repression of an anxiety-causing desire. The strong desire along with its related anxiety is then refocused from its original object to one which is symbolic. This symbolic fear then broadens in scope to include similar objects or places, until all of these items or places are feared and avoided. Freud originally conceived of this process as unfulfilled sexual tension. He believed that the energy accumulated in the repressed libido was ultimately discharged in a panic attack, and called his theory a "conversion reaction."

Freud first described this process in the case history of "Little Hans." Hans had a fear of horses which Freud attributed to an oedipal longing for his mother and fear of castration by his father. This anxiety-producing impulse was allegedly symbolically transferred to horses. (Hans's attacks began after he saw a horse's penis suddenly drop.) Freud discussed his theory with Hans's father and advised him to educate little Hans accordingly, but gently. Over a period of time, the boy eventually lost his fear of horses and was considered cured.

For Freud, therapeutic success came when the patient recognized his unconscious wishes, in other words, when the patient had developed "insight" into his problems. This was traditionally accomplished through a historical search of the patient's psychosexual background. In later years, Freud mellowed his viewpoint and acknowledged that patients would never be able to control their phobias simply by waiting for analysis to convince them to give them up.

Freud was the first to identify the importance of anxiety in mental disease. Throughout his career he continued to insist that anxiety was the central cause of most neuroses. He was not, however, the first to write about the subject. Fear and anxiety have always fascinated serious thinkers, and philosophers long before Freud's time studied their impact. Most experts believe that excessive pathological anxiety occurs as a result of trauma and involves intense feelings of helplessness.

As anxiety tends to take on a life of its own, it cannot be discharged from the nervous system. It may also stay attached to the memory of the original trauma or, in some cases, may be transferred to another object or exist as a free-floating sensation.

From a psychological point of view, anxiety cannot be released from the nervous system by the individual himself or through psy-

chotherapy or psychoanalysis. What has proved successful is prolonged exposure to the feared object, which ultimately causes
desensitization. The toleration of continuous fear for a few hours at
a time somehow allows the release of pent-up tensions and emotions.

The psychoanalytical theory began by defining anxiety as an intrapsychic problem (guilt and anxiety stemming from repressed sexual
desires)—a limited approach by anyone's standards. The theories
eventually were broadened to include environmental traumas, with
an emphasis on childhood and separation anxiety. With or without
the mother, a child is virtually helpless, and he recognizes that fact
very quickly. Helplessness means being unable to fulfill one's needs
and achieve satisfaction and a sense of security.

PSYCHOTHERAPY (INSIGHT THERAPY)

Psychotherapy is so well established in the Western world that any
criticism of its value is controversial at the very least. At the present
time, nearly 80 million people have sought its benefits at one time
or another. Furthermore, it's difficult to describe a therapy that has
at least 300 different variations. Almost any activity known to man
can be and probably has been labeled as "therapy." Sexual surrogate
therapy, work therapy, play therapy, exercise therapy, breathing ther-
apy, nude therapy, movie therapy, soap-opera therapy, pleasure
therapy, here-and-now therapy, historical therapy, and prelife therapy are all variations on this theme. The list is virtually endless.

Psychotherapy and the Common Cold

British researcher Hans J. Eysenck reported in 1952 that 72 percent
of a group of neurotic patients improved without treatment, while
only 44 percent improved with psychotherapy. This study, as you
can imagine, was soundly criticized, but it pointed up a number of
interesting questions. I remember reading an article in a 1961 British
publication which compared treatment by psychotherapy to treatment of the common cold. With treatment, it said, a cold will go
away in a week; without treatment, it will disappear in seven days.

Most neuroses generally disappear in about two years if untreated, but with psychotherapy, results take only twenty-four months! Or so some believe.

Insight Therapy

In spite of the numerous approaches to psychotherapy and the many major differences in philosophy and procedure, the results tend to be comparable. It appears that it is the general rather than specific aspects that produce changes. At the therapist's office, one can find compassion, concern, trust, and sanctuary. The patient expands his awareness and is encouraged to release and ventilate his emotions. He gets a clear, occasionally accurate explanation for his behavior, and that explanation helps fill another important need for a disturbed patient—the "need to know." Finally, the therapy provides the patient with another thing he greatly needs—an element of hope.

The purpose of insight therapy is to become aware of the processes going on in our subconcious minds. Once problems are identified, the patient continues to discuss his understanding over and over from many different points of view; through this process, he begins to experience a variety of emotions which evoke feelings about the past. Once emotional insight occurs, changes follow, causing the original symptoms to subside or disappear. At least, that's the theory behind the process, which at this point in time remains unproven.

Behavior Changes Before Insight

Some of us believe there are other possible explanations for the way changes occur, although this concept, too, is still in the theory stage. The reason some of us lean toward one explanation over another is that our particular beliefs seem to fit our own experiences more closely than do the concepts of other doctors. Many of us believe that *behavior changes occur prior to insights*, while the opposite holds true for those who believe that insight must come first.

In 1962 Dr. H. Hobbs was one of the first to suggest that behavioral changes occur prior to insight. In 1963 Dr. J. H. Cautela restated that theory in an articulate manner, asserting that learning the cause behind a particular problem does not necessarily change the problem, but altered behavior which resolves symptoms often allows the patient to connect these changes with the past. As patients were able to respond to a fearful situation in a new way, they found it possible to dredge up material from the past and discover its relationship to their present situation. In behavioral therapy, there is no deliberate attempt made to gather any past material.

BEHAVIORAL THERAPY

It is generally accepted that Joseph Wolpe started the behavioral therapy movement with his 1958 book *Psychotherapy by Reciprocal Inhibition* (Stanford University Press). From this simple beginning a wide variety of new techniques developed. I have listed those most frequently used.

Relaxation

This can be accomplished by gradual, conscious, controlled muscle relaxation, first propounded by E. Jacobson in *Progressive Relaxation* (1938). Another variation of this effective but time-consuming method is self-hypnosis. Both techniques are useful in the various phases of behavioral therapy. Biofeedback is the "high-tech" answer and can be equally effective in learning relaxation.

Reinforcement and Punishment

After a careful study of the patient in which occurrences before and after the undesired behavior are elicited, a program is set up that rewards good adaptive behavior. Maladaptive behavior is punished or in some way inhibited. Rewards can include praise or perks; punishment can be the loss of privileges.

Cognitive Therapy

An analysis is made of the way a patient groups his or her thoughts together to determine whether they are rational or irrational. The patient is trained to think more clearly, and negative-maladaptive thinking is replaced by thoughts that strengthen and encourage. For example, a patient suffering anxiety attacks may constantly be telling himself, "I'm going crazy." The person is asked instead to reaffirm: "I've never gone crazy yet, and I've been through this many times before." Or, "I have never been so sick that I've had to go to the hospital." Or, "My doctor says I'm merely anxious, not psychotic." When positive affirmations counter the negative thoughts, discomfort can begin to be minimized.

Exposure Therapy

This is another way of saying, "You have to face your fears." You can face them gradually, in a time-consuming process, or all at once, directly and more painfully, but with quicker results. Either way, the outcome is the same—you get better. Often relaxation or even medication is used to make the experience more tolerable; eventually, of course, these crutches must be discarded. The level of anxiety and the degree of resolve of the patient determine which approach is best: fast or slow. This is generally a successful approach.

Assertiveness Training

Some people have never learned how or have never desired to assert themselves with others. And they never will unless they discover how to take control and ask for what they want. Sometimes these patients lack social skills; they just don't know how to act effectively around other people, and inability to communicate causes them to become anxious. Through role playing and other techniques, these individuals are taught to behave and communicate differently, and they begin to experience different and more rewarding responses that lower their anxiety levels.

Aversion Therapy

This method, also known as shock therapy, involves giving a patient a painful electric shock whenever he thinks or does something that's forbidden. Normally, this type of therapy is used only as a last resort, in cases of addiction and serious sexual disorders. In one instance, a young man at a penal institution kept setting off the fire alarm. No amount of counseling seemed to deter him from his frequent (more than once a day) mischief. The psychiatrist finally applied electrodes to his head. They were attached to a portable battery box (an aversion device), and then he had his patient trigger the alarm at the same time he received a strong electric shock. After only two repetitions, the young man's behavior was corrected. Although extreme, aversion is sometimes the only treatment that will work.

IS HELPLESSNESS THE MAIN SOURCE OF ANXIETY?

It may sound strange to say that the mind and the body "talk to each other," but in essence they do. They communicate on a subconscious level, with the body telling the mind what it wants, how strongly it wants it, and how much energy it has available to put into the effort. The mind then assesses the environment and resources and tells the body what the chances are of achieving the desired goal. The emotions created from this interchange result from the power and quality of the need, and also the probability of fulfilling the need.

Fear is aroused when the mind uses internal and external cues to calculate whether or not it's going to be able to cope with the situation and achieve satisfaction, and then perceives it's going to fail—whether that need is to survive an attack, or to simply find food. Past experiences in similar situations lead us to decide whether or not we are capable of coping. It has been found that nervous or anxious people with low self-esteem often dramatically change and develop less anticipatory anxiety and less performance stress after their self-esteem has been raised effectively through therapy.

Most neurotics exercise little behavior control over the factors in a given situation. This happens because they *think* they have little control over anything that's related to their fears. It has also been recognized that neurotics use a particular strategy to think, acquire, and process information that is more impulsive than that of a normal individual. As we have said, it's your opinion of how you're doing, or how you *think* you can do, that so strongly affects your level of fear.

Many psychologists believe that some people learn how to be helpless by observing friends, acquaintances, or family members behaving in a helpless fashion. Others, including myself, believe that some people are genetically handicapped by a defect in their nor-adrenaline system so they do not have a normal resistance to stress. This is called the "motor activation defect theory." It implies that in some individuals a hereditary deficiency of noradrenaline comes to the fore when they are faced with a stress, especially one which they cannot avoid. Deficient individuals are only capable of a limited amount of activity, which is insufficient for learning and performing correct stress responses.

In one study, neurotics with many neurotic traits (those whose personal and hereditary histories lean strongly toward neuroses) had high anxiety levels. Those in the group with a lower level of neurotic traits (minimal personal or hereditary history indicating neuroses) had proportionately lower anxiety levels. The low-trait individuals, on stressful days, had relatively high noradrenaline levels, whereas the high-trait patients had a decrease in blood nor-adrenaline in similar situations. Identification of such biochemical imbalances has led to the reemergence of biological psychiatry.

REEMERGENCE OF BIOLOGICAL PSYCHIATRY

Prior to Freud, psychiatrists treated mental illness as they would any other physical disease. With Freud and his theories came talk therapy and different explanations as to the origins of psychological disturbances. But in the past five years or so, the newer understanding of how nerves transfer messages has led to a different view of anxiety and neuroses, and consequently treatment strategy has shifted back to physical approaches.

The Effects of Family Members on the Patient

There are times when patients don't wish to get better because they instinctively sense that if they improve, their relationship will suffer. In some instances, husbands have become impotent after their wives recovered from agoraphobia. A woman suddenly able to go where she pleases may make an insecure man fear that he has lost his power and control. Although the dependency relationship that results is quite disturbing to both parties, it can ultimately become a pattern from which the spouse derives some benefit.

In cases of abnormal jealousy in husbands of agoraphobics, therapy was less than normally effective, for such jealousy adversely affected the wives' response to treatment (Hafner 1979). Either husband or wife may deliberately create new problems such as "back trouble" in order to maintain similar balances in the relationship. If these changes and their effects on the husband are not taken seriously, therapy may be doomed.

Almost all research shows that spouses have very significant effects on patients and their symptoms. Patients whose marriages were unsatisfactory before treatment did not fare well during therapy, and they were likely to experience relapses after therapy was discontinued (Milton and Hafner 1979). The symptoms exhibited by the patients served to keep weak marriages from dissolving, and/or to protect spouses from self-examination of their own personality weaknesses. This illustrates the point that shaky marriages are not improved by getting people "better." Persons in such relationships are not necessarily made happier by conquering their disease. Destabilizing the tenuous balances may cause both parties to suffer more rather than less.

Agoraphobics and those with severe restrictive phobias are often accused of feigning sickness in order to manipulate others. In some cases this may be a factor, but the theory is generally refuted by research, and by most phobics themselves. The majority of agoraphobics are completely aware of the damage they are doing to themselves and others. Such individuals suffer humiliation and loneliness, and their personal suffering far exceeds any possible offsetting benefits.

At times a husband's need to be depended upon can become overwhelming; he may grow to derive great pleasure from being the "strong one" in the family. He may verbalize the desire for his wife to get better, but in actuality, he will in no way encourage her or push her in that direction. A husband's excessive emotional need for such dependency can reach pathological heights. In one case, after an agoraphobic patient made significant progress, the husband committed suicide.

How other family members of the agoraphobic patient respond

to inconveniences depends a lot on their finances as well as their characters. Well-adjusted and affluent families generally cope more easily with the restrictions imposed by a sick family member. But fewer options are available to families of limited economic resources, especially if they also contend with friction and instability. In such cases, the patient's problems tend to exacerbate an already difficult domestic situation.

The greater the patient's disability, the more need there is for the family to adapt to the problem. The deterioration of the patient that occurs over a long period of time, in some instances ten or more years, results in certain compensating balances within the family. Changes for the better in the ill partner often tend to unbalance a delicate situation. Research projects confirm that relatively sudden improvements in the patient will necessitate attitude changes and adjustments in the husband, children, or any other significant person in the patient's life (Hafner and Ross 1983). Besides the family's response to a patient's attempt to change, the patient's own attitude is critical. In cases where the patient was hypercritical of others and tended to blame others for his misery, change was less likely to occur.

In addition to certain negative underlying motivations of husbands to maintain control of their spouses, there are also other characteristics that interfere with treatment. Husbands who deny any anxiety about successful treatment of their wives will eventually destroy the patient's progress. While superficially these husbands may appear pleased, they may be experiencing discomfort and anxiety, which they don't even admit to themselves. These same husbands generally fail to give their wives emotional support during the critical phases of treatment, just when such help is desperately needed.

Such character observations should be factored into any treatment program. For example, spouses whose attitudes would interfere with progress should be helped to deal with their reluctance by being encouraged to take responsibility for their own problems. Joint family therapy or even individual therapy for the spouse is often useful. Any procedure that involves husbands and other family members and helps to reduce conflict will substantially contribute to the chances of success.

17

Health Problems Associated with Fears and Panic

Often organic problems are masked by anxiety and are consequently misdiagnosed, while other times, anxiety attacks occur as a result of physical disease and become a significant complication in the patient's illness. For example, anyone suffering a heart attack will also experience extreme anxiety, causing the release of toxic amounts of free fatty acids which are damaging to heart muscle. The anxiety must therefore be controlled as quickly as possible before it compounds the physical damage already in progress.

SOMATIZING ANXIETY (FROM MENTAL TO PHYSICAL)

It's been estimated that at least 20 billion dollars a year is spent in the treatment of people who are not diagnosed with a specific physical illness (Ford 1986). To "somatize" a mental disease means that the patient manifests physical symptoms of his mental disorder. There are a number of reasons why people sometimes want to pretend or believe that they are physically ill when there is little or no supportive evidence. Some individuals use illness as a means of gaining control or to divert attention from emotional conflicts. There are many more explanations, but in this instance we are interested chiefly in those who voice physical complaints as an alternative to facing emotional problems without being aware they are doing so. In other words, anxiety and depression are masked as physical complaints because in this form they may be less painful for the individual to accept and deal with. Most of the time such patients *are* truly unaware of what they are doing and firmly believe that their physical ailments are real. Because of the unconscious dynamics involved, simply confronting the patient with the truth does not help. If it were that simple, many forms of illness would be cured instantly. But unfortunately, an unconscious illness (neurosis) occurs for a specific reason, and the motivating "switch" is usually so strong that it prevents the individual from connecting with the truth.

It has been estimated that 5 percent of all patients who seek medical attention are suffering from major depression. If the depression has been switched (somatized) to a physical complaint such as headaches or sinusitis, then both the doctor and the patient are likely to pursue the wrong course of action. The patient rarely seems to make progress because the underlying disease frequently goes unrecognized and consequently untreated.

This book deals primarily with anxiety and how it is inextricably interwoven with physical symptoms. Disorders such as muscle aches and pains, fatigue, dizziness and light-headedness, breathlessness, chest pains, abdominal pains, sweating, choking, rapid heartbeats, and palpitations are only some of the physical complaints an anxiety patient can develop. The list is limitless.

What most often fools the doctor is having a patient complain of only a single symptom, such as chest pains. These complaints compel the doctor to search for an organic disease. Once tests prove negative, the patient is usually reassured that no disease is present, and the matter is concluded. But that doesn't stop the patient's worries, and his subsequent persistent, unrelenting complaints often convince the doctor that he is dealing with a hypochondriac. Only rarely will a physician question the patient thoroughly enough to uncover panic syndrome or anxiety problems.

A 1985 study by Laybourne and Redding provided data on twenty agoraphobic patients who were originally given incorrect diagnoses, such as "sexual conflict," hypoglycemia, alcoholism, or general "nervousness." One of the patients even suggested agoraphobia to her physician but was ignored. Instead, after an electroencephalogram (EEG), lumbar puncture, brain scan, and X rays, she was diagnosed as having "dizziness of unknown origin." Most patients with anxiety disorders are not able to make their own diagnoses and usually do not volunteer enough information unless specifically encouraged by an interested and enlightened physician.

Anxiety Following Viral Infections

It has been found that depression sometimes develops in patients recovering from infectious mononucleosis (Codie and Nye 1976). Many reports confirm these findings regarding the Epstein-Barr virus. If depression and anxiety accompanied by psychological malaise come quickly after or along with the active viral infection, then physicians seldom have difficulty determining the source of anxiety and/or depression. On the other hand, there may be a recovery period before the infectious agent transforms itself from an acute disease to a chronic one. This chronic viremia, in addition to causing fatigue, can alter the personality so that one is depressed or anxious all the time. It may even lead to a histrionic type of personality. Any chronic illness may start to modify the personality so that the victim becomes different. Previously strong, independent people become hypochondriacal and emotional, often much more cautious and frightened than they had been previously (Allen and Tilkian 1986).

Hypoglycemia

Many readers are already aware of hypoglycemia (low blood sugar). But the symptoms, if severe, may sometimes be confused with anxiety attacks. Although the manifestations of hypoglycemia are similar to panic syndrome, they can be differentiated.

SYMPTOMS INCLUDE:

Anxiety	Confusion
Tremors	Double vision
Palpitations	Clumsiness
Rapid heartbeat	Personality changes
Sweating	Difficulty in thinking
Weakness	Depression
Hunger	Lethargy
Headaches	

You can see how similar these symptoms are to those of panic disorders. In some cases, acute anxiety may actually cause people to become hypoglycemic, although research has not been conclusive. It should, however, be noted that chronic stress with secondary anxiety has been linked to the onset of hypoglycemia, perhaps due to the repeated reactive release of adrenaline in response to repetitive stress situations.

The brain is the most sensitive organ in the body and highly vulnerable to a decrease in blood sugar because it requires a constant supply of carbohydrates. The hypothalamus, the part of the brain that exerts extensive control over the involuntary nervous system, is also sensitive to hypoglycemia. The involuntary nervous system symptoms which result from the release of adrenaline do, in some ways, masquerade as the symptoms of panic disorders.

Because neurological damage can occur from untreated hypoglycemia, diagnosis is important, and, fortunately, relatively simple. The five-hour glucose tolerance test is frequently used to determine hypoglycemia as well as diabetes. Although there is some dispute over how to read the results clearly, the test as a whole is reliable. A second method, less scientific in nature, is to provide the patient with food while he is experiencing anxiety symptoms. Relief of anxiety will usually occur rapidly, especially if the food received is a carbohydrate. Some hypoglycemics foolishly use stimulants such as caffeine and nicotine to "treat" their condition, but these substances have a negative rather than a mitigating effect.

Generally, some symptom relief can be obtained by avoiding alcohol, refined carbohydrates, caffeine, and cigarettes. A sound diet also makes a positive difference, as do more frequent meals and moderate but frequent use of salt.

Vasovagal Syncopy

Vasovagal syncopy is an acute fall in blood pressure due to massive relaxation of peripheral blood vessels. Caused by pain or fear, it results in an extremely fast heartbeat or unconsciousness and occasionally convulsions if oxygen in the brain is extreme. In susceptible individuals, any sudden excitement may cause a pooling of large amounts of blood in the dilated blood vessels in the muscles. The blood may be unable to leave the muscle because the veins, which permit the blood to return to the heart, are obstructed from muscle tension and thus blocked. Not enough blood can get back to the heart, causing the heart rate to decrease and thus deprive the brain of needed blood and oxygen. The patient may feel light-headed, dizzy, or faint. These symptoms will occur more rapidly if he is standing or sitting, because gravity also acts to keep blood from the brain.

One of the benefits of benzodiazepines (tranquilizers) is that they stop the reaction to both pain and fear. They are therefore of benefit to patients with this illness. Most pain medications will block pain but do not affect the relaxation reflex of blood vessels caused by trauma, and so they are less helpful to these patients.

Pheochromocytoma

A tumor on the adrenal gland called a pheochromocytoma may cause symptoms that sometimes resemble those of anxiety and panic patients. Many of these tumors go unrecognized during the life of the patient and are discovered only during autopsies. They occur in about one out of every 1,000 people in general. Unlike hypogly-cemia, this disease is more difficult to differentiate from panic syn-drome, and cases of misdiagnosis have frequently been reported.

SYMPTOMS INCLUDE:

Rapid heartbeat	Breathing difficulties
Palpitations	Headaches
Trembling	Unusual flushing or paleness

Sudden movements can trigger anxiety attacks in patients with pheochromocytoma, and another common manifestation is throb-bing headaches. Neither of these symptoms is commonly seen in persons with panic syndrome, but only special tests will accurately diagnose the disease.

An Overactive Thyroid Gland— Thyrotoxicosis

Many of the symptoms seen in patients with an overactive thyroid gland are also found in those with high levels of anxiety. Naturally, any highly anxious patient should be screened for thyroid disease to avoid misdiagnosis.

SYMPTOMS INCLUDE:

Nervousness	Eye problems
Sensitivity to heat	Weight loss
Fatigue	Weakness
Rapid heartbeat	Increased appetite
Excessive sweating	Breathing difficulties
Palpitations	Diarrhea or bowel complaints

As you can see, these symptoms are indistinguishable from those of anxiety patients, but there are certain symptoms that do separate the two diseases. Overactive thyroid patients generally feel tired, but continue to function, while anxiety patients often become immobilized. Another difference to note is that thyroid patients have good circulation in the hands, evidenced by warmness, while the anxiety patient has cold, clammy hands. The overactive thyroid patient always has a rapid pulse, while the anxiety patient may have a slower pulse when relaxed or asleep. Interestingly, both conditions can be treated by the same drug, propranolol.

Raynaud's Syndrome

A constriction of the blood vessels of both hands and feet causes severely limited circulation. The temperature of these areas drops so that the hands and feet feel chilled even in warm weather. Their color often becomes blue or purple and eventually white if not enough blood reaches the area. These changes are periodic and occur in response to cold weather, exercise, and emotional changes. If the disease occurs at an early age, there can be a significant underdevelopment of the hands and feet. Although the cause is not fully known, it is suspected to result from a defect in the local blood vessels of the extremities.

There have been reported cases of depression and panic disorders occurring in association with Raynaud's Syndrome (Mueller and Allen 1984). There are also connections between Raynaud's Syndrome, panic syndrome, and periodic depression, because all three groups often report lower than normal temperatures in the extremities. All three may produce this problem in the same way, by activating what are called the *alpha-receptors*. These receptors are sensitive spots on blood vessels which, if activated, constrict the vessels. Drugs that block alpha-receptor sensitivity have been used in treatment (tolazoline for Raynaud's and clonidine for panic disorders). A relationship exists between these diseases, but there has not yet been extensive investigation.

Epilepsy

As far back as 1956, reports have appeared linking epilepsy with episodes of depression, anxiety, or fear (Weil 1956). Such theories are based on the fact that epileptic seizures can originate in various locations in the brain near emotional centers. Those patients whose seizure source occurs near an area of the brain responsible for emotions may experience emotions along with other forms of seizures or they may simply feel "seizures of emotion." In other words, the actual seizure comes in the form of a panic attack.

Such cases have been illustrated in medical literature (Herman and Chhabria 1980). Herman and Chhabria reported two examples of young adults with histories of epilepsy since childhood. They experienced fear before each seizure, then began having panic attacks even without seizures, as the attacks took on a life of their own. Brain studies during those episodes demonstrated *epileptiform* brain waves. In both cases the area of disturbance was near or in the amygdala, an area of the brain known to be associated with emotions.

In the first case, the twenty-year-old female said she felt "as though I'm going to be hit by a car—a terrifying feeling—other times it feels as if someone is in the room waiting to attack me. I'm so scared I run and hide—sometimes under my bed. I'm frightened to death." Because it is human nature to need desperately to understand what is happening, if no explanation is available, the victim will invent one. In this case, as in the one to follow, the patient would suddenly experience panic and then associate it with anyone who might be present. Often she would flee from the person and run to a "safe" place. In the beginning she recognized her irrationality, but once the fear was unleashed, she could not control her behavior.

The second case involved a twenty-two-year-old male with a similar history, who described his feelings as "nightmarish—a feeling of doom—like death." In both instances, as the panic seizures occurred more often, the patients began to believe that these feelings must be "real," that they were really faced with an actual danger.

In each case, the individual was not able to cope with these sudden attacks which came from out of the blue, and both began to exhibit bizarre behavior. The young woman withdrew from others and stayed in places she considered safe. Eventually she began to threaten strangers as she developed delusions of imminent danger. The young man would hide in police stations or he would board himself up in his room. He eventually began ransacking other persons' apartments searching for evidence of a "plot" to harm him.

The constant unexplained fears began to overwhelm their victims, and slowly to warp their reasoning and behavior. Both became increasingly paranoid as the unrelenting attacks of fear persisted. Their plight demonstrates the power of uncontrolled emotions to alter and shape beliefs and thought patterns so profoundly that retraining, even if possible, is excruciatingly difficult.

While these two cases clearly demonstrate the early association of panic attacks and seizures, it is possible for the panic attacks to come without the accompaniment of seizures. There have been similar theories related to bulimia, indicating that an eating binge might possibly be a form of seizure. Although only a small percentage of panic patients fall into this category, the possibility of epilepsy should be considered before a final diagnosis is made.

It has been reported that more than half of those who exhibited seizures also experienced some form of fear or depression. Usually those expressing fear had abnormal electrical discharges from areas of the brain nearest the temples. Research more than twenty-five years ago noted that stimulation of the *amygdaloid nucleus* in animals produces fear. Part of this amygdaloid area is located near the temples where epileptic seizures often originate.

Fear exhibited by most epileptics may vary from slight to intense and sometimes progresses to a state of complete terror. The symptoms persist for a different length of time in each individual. In addition to feelings of panic, epileptics, like agoraphobics, often experience breathlessness, nausea and vomiting with abdominal pain or discomfort, palpitations, rapid heartbeat, gooseflesh, sweating, and all of the phenomena associated with the involuntary nervous system. Actual phobias related to certain places or events can also develop. These phobias may or may not actually occur during or near the time of a seizure, but they are definitely part of this complex illness.

Serotonin-Irritation Syndrome

It appears that positively charged air (positive ions) can increase the neurotransmitter serotonin in the brain. When this occurs, the sensitive patient becomes irritable. Studies have clearly indicated that the behavior of insects and animals can be changed when the concentration of positively or negatively charged air (negative ions) is altered. Positive-charged ions seem to create anxiety in animals, and these increases in anxiety have been related to increases in brain serotonin. The disorder is now considered to be an authentic medical entity, both diagnosable and treatable.

Changes in the weather, winds in particular, are the responsible agents in determining whether the air will be more positively or more negatively inclined. Electrical equipment, especially high-tension power lines, also appears to positively charge surrounding air. When these charged particles increase the serotonin level in the brain, an individual may feel irritable or anxious and might experience nausea, vomiting, and diarrhea.

Increased serum serotonin can be determined with lab tests and may be used to contribute to a complete diagnosis. There are companies that now manufacture negative-ion generators. These relatively inexpensive devices can be helpful to those who suffer from such sensitivities. Methysergide, 2 mg twice daily, has also been found to alleviate these symptoms.

Hyperventilation Syndrome

This is a well-known and rather common condition, with symptoms which are again similar to those of panic disorders. Patients have a tendency to overbreathe, and the resulting hyperventilation causes the blood to become alkaline, which in turn lowers the oxygen level in the brain, resulting in all of the following symptoms:

Visual disturbances	Dizziness
Confusion	Ringing in the ears
Disturbed consciousness	Numbness in the fingers and
Faintness	around the mouth

A milder form produces symptoms as follows:

| Chronic clearing the throat | Yawning |
| Constant sniffling | Sighing |

You can see how the symptoms might be confused with a panic attack. We have dealt with this subject in more detail in other chapters.

Mitral Valve Prolapse

Harold is a thirty-year-old-mechanic, a bachelor, and a seemingly healthy young man, who suffers from chest pains. He has something in common with his neighbor Elizabeth, who has palpitations and a fluttering heart which sometimes leads to arrhythmia. Both of these relatively young people have a very old disease with a new name: It's called *mitral valve prolapse.*

A hundred years ago, a young lady whose heart fluttered was said to have an "irritable" heart, that is, if it wasn't just a simple case of being "in love." During the First World War, men who experienced these symptoms were diagnosed as having a "soldier's heart" or *neurocirculatory asthenia.* In the Second World War, the label was "anxiety neurosis."

Mitral valve prolapse means that a valve in the heart is defective, and the cause is usually genetic in origin. As much as 7 percent of the total population has this condition but often without symptoms. It is the most common disease of the valves of the heart in Western countries.

This condition involves a redundancy of valve tissue which allows blood to pass in the wrong direction between two chambers of the heart. When the heart contracts, blood is supposed to be expelled into the arteries and on to the rest of the body. The mitral valve prevents the blood from going backward in the heart. When there is extra tissue and looseness of this valve, it incorrectly billows backwards with the pressure of the contracting heart. This may reduce the amount of blood going to the body, since some of the blood is going into the billowing valve in the opposite direction of its proper route.

Mitral valve prolapse alone does not generally produce panic attacks, but may act as a trigger in patients who already have the disorder. It has also been suggested that both types of patients may have a common pathology, namely a disturbance of the involuntary nervous system.

COMMON CHARACTERISTICS

Mitral Valve Prolapse	*Anxiety Disorders*
Predominantly females	Predominantly females
Onset before age 40	Onset before age 40
Found in 2–10 percent of the population	Found in 2–20 percent of the population
Genetic links	Genetic links

Many of those with mitral valve prolapse have frequent transient, unexplainable rises in the levels of adrenalinelike substances in their blood, especially during daylight hours. All of the instigators are not known, but caffeine, stressful situations, increased activity, and rapid changes in body position and posture can all be contributing factors.

As a cause of anxiety, we have discussed increased adrenergic tone. Many consider this to be partially responsible for a number of symptoms. Studies have verified that patients with mitral valve prolapse also show increased resting tone to their adrenergic system, and are hypersensitive to adrenal stimulation. This group of individuals often has a low tolerance to exercise, so treadmill tests should be used judiciously in diagnosis.

Many, if not most, patients with mitral valve prolapse show no symptoms, and the defect is usually detected only during a physical examination. On the other hand, at some point in the victim's life, usually around the age of thirty, the symptoms described below may begin to appear. In a few people, they may become quite severe. The symptoms of mitral valve prolapse syndrome include anxiety, an exhaustive type of fatigue, rapid and irregular heartbeat, difficulty breathing, chest pains, dizziness, numbness around the mouth and in the hands, low blood pressure, and sometimes panic attacks, all caused by the involuntary nervous system. Other associated manifestations include migraine and sleep disorders.

Breathlessness, fatigue, dizziness, and anxiety are not pleasant, but they aren't in themselves dangerous. Sometimes, however, they can lead to conditions which are life-threatening. A German medical journal reported that young adults with fears of heart disease (cardiophobia) may develop circulatory problems. Besides mitral valve prolapse, they may experience temporary episodes of decreased circulation (ischemia) in either the heart or the brain. The journal goes on to advise that doctors should take seriously all adults, especially young adults, who complain of fears of heart disease. They suggest echocardiography and serial electrocardiogram (ECG) examinations as a precautionary measure. Interest in this disease rose when research studies reported that nearly a third of all anxiety patients concurrently suffered from mitral valve prolapse.

Cardiac performance was evaluated in 194 children with symptomatic mitral valve prolapse, using the isometric hand-grip test. All patients showed an abnormal response to hand grip before treatment. Eight children received 2 mg/kg/day of co-enzyme Q10 (CoQ10) for eight weeks, and eight received a placebo. Hand-grip tests became normal in seven of the CoQ10-treated patients, and in none of the placebo patients. Relapse frequently occurred in patients who stopped the medication within twelve to seventeen months, but was rarely seen in those who took CoQ10 for eighteen months or more. Co-enzyme Q-10 ubiquinone, a naturally occurring molecule similar to vitamin K, is important in the formation of energy.

Magnesium deficiency has been associated with this syndrome also and could account for many, if not all, of the symptoms produced. Durlock (1981) claims that symptoms were controlled in a third of the patients who were treated with magnesium during a one-year period. A magnesium deficiency tends to increase circulatory adrenaline and predisposes the patient to heart irregularities and deregulation of the voluntary nervous system. The disturbance in these systems can easily explain why these patients have symptoms similar to panic patients. Magnesium therapy has been found to eliminate mitral valve prolapse symptoms, especially when augmented by essential fatty acids (Gabland, Baker, and McLellan 1986). A treatment that has proven useful for symptomatic patients is 100 mg magnesium lactate three times daily, along with capsules of essential fatty acids, three to six daily.

Irritable Bowel Syndrome

There are reported cases of patients appearing in doctors' offices complaining of gastrointestinal disturbances but who, on closer examination, are actually suffering from an underlying anxiety disorder. Their original complaints were of cramping, constipation, or diarrhea. As further confirmation of this phenomenon, studies on psychiatric patients demonstrate a high percentage of patients with functional bowel problems similar to those listed above. Even more convincing is that studies on patients first diagnosed as suffering from irritable bowel syndrome show that as much as 70 to 90 percent of them have diagnosable mental health problems—especially anxiety and depression.

It has been concluded by one research group that some panic disorder patients may seek help first for gastrointestinal symptoms instead of panic (Lydiard and Laraia 1986). In fact, for these patients, panic disorder and irritable bowel syndrome may be the same illness. The proof of the pudding is that irritable-bowel-syndrome patients often respond more favorably when treated for anxiety and depression than when treated for an irritable bowel.

TMJ—Temporomandibular Joint Syndrome Anxiety

There seems to be no end to the "odd" causes for anxiety, almost as many causes as there are people. In a case reported by Stan and McGrath (1984), a twenty-year-old female developed anxiety and tension along with a TMJ condition after a negative experience with a general anesthetic. People often emerge from general anesthesia in a state of excitement, usually short-lived. It has been reported that the same phenomenon may occur in patients aroused from cardiac bypasses, and, again, the symptoms usually disappear. But in some instances, as in the above case, they may persist and eventually require treatment for the anxiety.

Summary

This list of anxiety-related diseases is not complete, but there are enough examples for you to get an overview of the problem.

Anxiety is one of the major symptoms of a variety of diseases. This may lead to confusion as to whether anxiety is the cause or the result of an accompanying physical illness. Doctors and patients must be alert to these relationships in order to determine proper treatment. I emphasize this point because misdiagnoses of anxiety attacks, agoraphobia, and depression are extremely common, as is demonstrated in medical literature. As a reader of this book, your awareness of this possibility will help you work with your physician toward a complete and accurate diagnosis so that you can receive the best possible treatment.

18

Getting Further Help

SOME FINAL POINTS RELATED TO NUTRITIONAL SUPPLEMENTS

To gain maximum benefit from this book and to control your fears effectively using nutritional supplements, keep the following thoughts in mind.

You're an Individual

At first glance, we humans all look pretty similar, but on closer inspection, there are countless differences. In each of us, the bio-chemical-physical makeup is totally unique. No two humans are exactly alike.

The nutrients that effectively diminish fears will differ from one person to the next. You must search for your own special formula by changing the supplements until you're satisfied. How many times have you heard people say, "Oh, I tried that but it didn't work," and when you inquired how many times they tried, you were told, "Oh, once or twice"? It probably will take more than a couple of attempts to be successful.

Some people act as though they're helpless; they make a pitifully small effort and then quit if there's no one around to encourage them. I hope *you* are going to do a lot better than that.

You Can Do It

Nutritional supplements are highly effective in blocking anxiety and fear. With practice you can become an expert. You don't need a degree in biochemistry to control fears. You need to use your head to figure out what is right for you. You need to spend a little time on trial and error. My experience has shown that most people can find an effective remedy if they are patient.

Circumstances Are Unique

Was there ever a time in your life when one event was identical to another? Of course not. Sometimes we think we experience *déjà vu*, but in actuality, life doesn't repeat itself.

A formula that works well at one time may not succeed at another. With all of the suggestions found in this book, you'll have more than enough alternatives to work with in case you should develop a tolerance to one set of supplements and it should no longer be effective in helping you.

Time Marches On

The human shape is essentially dynamic. It changes over the years. First we grow tall, then females develop curves, males build heavier muscles, and those who aren't careful can grow "forward" with middle-age spread. Finally, we grow shorter with advanced age. If we suffer glandular disease, we may also change in other ways. Our body chemistry balance, too, is subject to fluctuation. These patterns lead to new responses to nutrients. From time to time you may need to recompute your set of supplements and tailor them to your body's needs at that particular time.

Anxiety Can Be the Symptom of a More Serious Disease

Anxiety or fear can be symptomatic of a mild or severe imbalance of homeostasis causing a person's whole system to get off kilter. It can also indicate serious disease. If you suspect that you suffer from an underlying ailment, you may need professional help. You might get in touch with the organizations listed in this chapter or seek additional consultation.

The Message of This Book

Throughout this book I have stressed the combined effect of proper nutrition and behavioral modification of the body's functioning and the value of nutritional supplements in relieving symptoms. Nutrition alone, however, has its limitations, for it doesn't encourage personal growth. For that you need to combat your fears through experiences that increase your understanding as well as your ability to cope.

You can achieve growth by yourself through self-help methods, or you can grow with the assistance of others. In either case, the second part of your program must involve a deliberate effort to face your fears. I have recommended numerous self-help methods that will aid you in dissipating your fears, methods that have already been proven successful in research studies. If you skillfully follow directions, you too will begin to change as your fears diminish. If, on the other hand, you choose to combine the assistance of the nutritional supplements listed in this book with professional help, I have listed some sources below.

A Place to Find Help

The National Self-Help Clearinghouse maintains an up-to-date listing of most mutual-aid organizations throughout the nation. You will need to send a stamped self-addressed envelope.

National Self-Help Clearinghouse
City University of New York
33 West 42nd St.
New York, New York 10036
212-840-1259

Local numbers for support groups:

	Self Help
CALIFORNIA	800-222-LINK
CONNECTICUT	203-789-7645
ILLINOIS	312-328-0470
KANSAS	316-686-1205
MICHIGAN	616-983-7781
MINNESOTA	612-925-0585
NEBRASKA	402-476-9668
NEW JERSEY	201-625-9565
NEW YORK STATE	518-695-3418
NEW YORK CITY	212-788-8787
OHIO	216-696-4262
OREGON	503-222-5555
PENNSYLVANIA	215-568-0890 Ext. 266

If air travel is your problem, contact

Institute for Psychology of Air Travel
Massachusetts Psychological Center
25 Huntington Ave.
Boston, MA 02116
(617) 437-1811

You might also phone the nearest major airport for a reference. Doctors who belong to the organizations listed in this chapter are generally knowledgeable about the effects of allergies on emotions and have usually attended seminars and conferences on the subject. They read the journals related to clinical ecology and allergy and have experience with such patients. However, there may be some who do not have an interest or special expertise in these subjects, so be selective when you use the recommendations and interview two or three physicians before making a decision.

Professional Organizations Related to Allergy, Nutrition, and Preventive Medicine

American College of
  Advancement in Medicine
23121 Verdugo Dr. #204
Laguna Hills, CA 92653

International College of
  Applied Nutrition
P.O. Box 286
La Habra, CA 90631

Price Potenger Foundation
P.O. Box 2614
La Mesa, CA 92041

The Orthomolecular Medical
  Society
6151 West Century Blvd.
Los Angeles, CA 90045

American Academy of
  Environmental Medicine
P.O. Box 16106
Denver, CO 80216

American Academy of
  Otolaryngic Allergy
1101 Vermont Ave., NW #302
Washington, DC 20005

Human Ecology Action League
505 N. Lakeshore Drive, #6505
Chicago, IL 60611

International Academy of
  Preventative Medicine
P.O. Box 25276
Shawnee Mission, KS 66225

Academy of Orthomolecular
  Psychiatry
1691 Northern Blvd.
Manhasset, NY 11031

INTERNATIONALLY

Holistic Practitioner Network
17 Randle St.
Sunny Hills, Australia 20010

Other Information Sources: Related to Allergy and Nutrition

Access to Nutritional Data
P.O. Box 52
Ashby, MA 01431

Human Ecology Action League
  (HEAL)
7330 N. Rojers Ave.
Chicago, IL 60626

Center for Science in the Public
  Interest
1501 16th St. NW
Washington, DC 20036

AMINO-ACID ANALYSIS

Amino-acid analysis may be done with the help of a physician. The Atron Company in Santa Monica will provide a list of the doctors in your general area who do the analysis.

Atron Company
1661 Lincoln Blvd. #300
Santa Monica, CA 90404

ORGANIZATIONS THAT DEAL WITH PMS

Hunt Medical Group
3808 Riverside Drive
North Hollywood, CA 91602

PMS Center
9201 Sunset Blvd.
Los Angeles, CA 90069

PMS Connection
Women's Medical Center
5985 W. Pico Blvd.
Los Angeles, CA 90035

PMS Treatment Center
150 N. Santa Anita
Arcadia, CA 91006

*Premenstrual Syndrome
   Consultants of Colorado*
6415 W. 44th St.
Wheatridge, CO 80033

PMS Community Awareness
1914 Chandler Lane
Columbus, IN 47203

Dr. Michelle Harrison
763 Massachusetts Ave.
Cambridge, MA 02139

PMS Research Foundation
P.O. Box 14574
Las Vegas, NV 89114

PMS Medical Group
140 West End Ave.
New York, NY 10023

National PMS Society
P.O. Box 11467
Durham, NC 27703

Family and Teen Health Services
Green County Memorial Hospital
Waynesburg, PA 15370

PMS Action, Inc.
P.O. Box 9326
Madison, WI 53715

BULIMIA AND ANOREXIA

American Anorexia/Bulimia
  Association, Inc.
133 Cedar Lane
Teaneck, NJ 07666
(201) 836-1800

National Anorexia Aid Society
P.O. Box 29461
Columbia, OH 43229
(614) 846-6810

National Association of Anorexia
  & Associated Disorders
Box 271
Highland Park, IL 60035
(312) 831-3438

SLEEP DISORDER ORGANIZATIONS

American Narcolepsy
  Association, Inc.
1139 Bush St., Suite D
San Carlos, CA 94070-2477
(415) 591-7979

American Narcolepsy Association
P.O. Box 5846
Stanford, CA 94305
(415) 591-7979

Miscellaneous

National Alliance for the
  Mentally Ill
1200 15th St., NW
Washington, DC 20005
(202) 833-3530

Association for Children and
  Adults with Learning
  Disabilities
4156 Library Rd.
Pittsburgh, PA 15234
(412) 341-1515

Epilepsy Foundation of America
4351 Garden City Drive
Landover, MD 20785
(301) 459-3700

A WORD ABOUT PROFESSIONAL HELP

Psychiatrists

It might seem strange to be referred to a psychiatrist for help in using a nutritional program, but there's a reason for it. Psychiatrists are often at the forefront of innovative ideas, and such assistance may be necessary if your problems are acute. Many psychiatrists belong to the preventive medicine associations listed in this chapter. You may get their addresses from these organizations.

Psychologists and Social Workers

Usually these two groups are better trained in behavioral therapy than most physicians. Each one has a different skill level, but they are excellent sources for bringing about change, and most are very open to combining their therapy with nutritional supplements.

Clinical Ecologists

Most doctors in this group have spent a good deal of time and money training in this specialty. They understand all phases of neurological allergies and mental illness and have probably treated dozens of cases such as yours. But there is just one problem: there are too many people with health problems and too few clinical ecologists. Most doctors in this group have backgrounds in allergies, internal medicine, or psychiatry and are well equipped to assist you, but in spite of their short supply, be as selective as you can.

Nutritionists

There are many good nutritionists in private practice who can dispense knowledgeable information. Though nutritionists offer valuable services, remember that they can't write prescriptions, so you may need to consult a physician and be under his care simultaneously if your fears and anxieties are severe enough to require medication.

The Family Doctor

If nutritional changes alone aren't enough, you might seek the cooperation of a physician. But don't expect to walk into a doctor's office and ask for a prescription without his or her evaluation. Doctors aren't pharmacists; they must decide whether it's wise or unwise to prescribe medications for a particular ailment. They also require assurances that drugs won't be abused. The overuse of drugs is a major problem in today's society and some of the drugs used to control anxiety can fall into this category.

It may be difficult for patients troubled by anxiety and fear to find general practitioners who are oriented to a non-drug approach. Only a few family physicians belong to the organizations listed above. Others, unfortunately, may not be helpful, unless you wish to take medication only for your symptoms.

Female Physicians

For some reason I have found women to be more open to new ideas than men—or at least it seems so in medicine. A female physician may be the right person to see, especially if she specializes in the proper use of nutrition.

Summary

If the sources listed above are not totally satisfactory, then ask for a referral, and go from there. The chief idea is not to be helpless. Your life and your health can be changed, but not without your input. You are not helpless unless you decide to be. You are not the victim unless you let yourself be. With proper nutrition and a good plan for therapy, you've stacked the deck in your favor. You now have the power to change. So go to it, and keep on growing—for the rest of your life.

APPENDIX

APPENDIX

PHOBIAS

Air or heights	Aerophobia	Choking	Pnigophobia
Animals	Zoophobia	Cholera	Cholerophobia
Bacteria	Bacteriophobia	Churches	Ecclesiaphobia
Beards	Phgonophobia	Clothing	Vestiophobia
Beds	Clinophobia	Clouds	Nephophobia
Bees	Apiphobia	Cold	Psychrophobia
Being afraid	Phobophobia	Colors	Chromatophobia
Being alone	Autophobia	Confined in a	
Being beaten	Rhabdophobia	house	Domatophobia
Being bound	Merinthophobia	Corpses	Necrophobia
Being buried		Crossing a bridge	Gephyrophobia
alive	Taphephobia	Crowds	Ochlophobia
Being dirty	Automysophobia	Crystals	Crystallophobia
Being egotistical	Autophobia	Dampness	Hygrophobia
Being scratched	Amychophobia	Darkness	Achluophobia
Being stared at	Scopophobia	Dawn	Eosophobia
Birds	Ornithophobia	Daylight	Phengophobia
Blood	Hematophobia	Dead bodies	Necrophobia
Blushing	Erythrophobia	Death	Thanatophobia
Books	Bibliophobia	Deformity	Dysmorphophobia
Cancer	Cancerophobia	Demons	Demonophobia
Cats	Ailurophobia	Depths	Bathophobia
Certain names	Onomatophobia	Dirt	Mysophobia
Childbirth	Tocophobia	Disease	Nosophobia
Children	Pediophobia	Disorder	Ataxiophobia
China	Sinophobia	Doctors	Iatrophobia

Dogs	Cynophobia	Graves	Taphophobia
Dolls	Pediophobia	Gravity	Barophobia
Drafts	Anemophobia	Hair	Trichophobia
Dreams	Oncirophobia	Hair	Chaetophobia
Drink	Potophobia	Heart disease	Cardiophobia
Drinking	Dipsophobia	Heat	Thermophobia
Drugs	Pharmacophobia	Heaven	Uranophobia
Duration	Chronophobia	Heights	Acrophobia
Dust	Amathophobia	Heredity	Patriophobia
Electricity	Electrophobia	Home	Domatophobia
Elevated places,		Home	
heights	Acrophobia	surroundings	Ecophobia
Empty rooms	Kenophobia	Horses	Hippophobia
Enclosed space	Claustrophobia	Human beings	Anthropophobia
England and		Ice, frost	Cryophobia
things English	Anglophobia	Ideas	Ideophobia
Everything	Pantophobia	Illness	Nosophobia
Eyes	Ommatophobia	Imperfection	Atelophobia
Failure	Kakorraphiaphobia	Infection	Mysophobia
Fatigue	Ponophobia	Infinity	Apeirophobia
Feces	Coprophobia	Inoculation,	
Fire	Pyrophobia	injections	Trypanophobia
Fish	Ichthyophobia	Insanity	Lyssophobia
Flashes	Selaphobia	Insanity	Dementophobia
Flogging	Mastigophobia	Insects	Entomophobia
Flood	Antlophobia	Itching	Acarophobia
Flowers	Anthophobia	Jealousy	Zelophobia
Flutes	Aulophobia	Justice	Dikephobia
Flying	Aviophobia	Knees	Genuphobia
Fog	Homichlophobia	Lakes	Limnophobia
Food	Sitophobia	Learning	Sophophobia
Foreigners	Xenophobia	Left side	Levophobia
France and		Leprosy	Leprophobia
things French	Gallophobia	Light	Photophobia
Fur	Doraphobia	Lightning	Astraphobia
Gaiety	Cherophobia	Machinery	Mechanophobia
Germany and		Making decisions	Decidophobia
things German	Germanophobia	Making false	
Germs	Spermophobia	statements	Mythophobia
Ghosts	Phasmophobia	Many things	Polyphobia
Glass	Crystallophobia	Marriage	Gamophobia
God	Theophobia	Meat	Carnophobia
Going to bed	Clinophobia	Men	Androphobia

Metals	Metallophobia	Pregnancy	Maieusiophobia
Meteors	Meteorophobia	Punishment	Poinephobia
Mice	Musophobia	Rabies	Lyssophobia
Microbes	Bacilliphobia	Railways	Siderodromophobia
Mind	Psychophobia	Rain	Ombrophobia
Mirrors	Eisoptrophobia	Reptiles	Herpetophobia
Missiles	Ballistophobia	Responsibility	Hypegiaphobia
Moisture	Hygrophobia	Ridicule	Katagelophobia
Money	Chrometophobia	Rivers	Potamophobia
Monstrosities	Teratophobia	Robbers	Harpaxophobia
Motion	Kinesophobia	Ruin	Atephobia
Moving or making changes	Tropophobia	Russia or things Russian	Russophobia
Nakedness	Gymnophobia	Rust	Iophobia
Names	Nomatophobia	Sacred things	Hierophobia
Narrowness	Anginaphobia	Satan	Satanophobia
Needles and pins	Belonophobia	School	Scholionophobia
Neglect of duty	Paralipophobia	Sea	Thalassophobia
Negroes	Negrophobia	Sea swell	Cymophobia
New	Neophobia	Sex	Genophobia
Night	Nyctophobia	Sexual intercourse	Coitophobia
Noise or loud talking	Phonophobia	Shadows	Sciophobia
Novelty	Cenophobia	Sharp objects	Belonophobia
Numbers	Numerophobia	Shock	Hormephobia
Odors (body)	Osphresiophobia	Sinning	Peccatophobia
Odors	Osmophobia	Sitting idle	Thaasophobia
One thing	Monophobia	Skin	Dermatophobia
Oneself	Autophobia	Skin of animals	Doraphobia
One's own fears	Phobophobia	Sleep	Hypnophobia
Open spaces	Agoraphobia	Smell	Olfactorphobia
Pain	Algophobia	Smothering	Pnigerophobia
Parasites	Parasitophobia	Snakes	Ophidiophobia
Particular places	Topophobia	Snow	Chionophobia
People	Anthropophobia	Society	Anthropophobia
Physical love	Erotophobia	Solitude	Eremophobia
Plants	Botanophobia	Sound	Akousticophobia
Pleasure	Hedonophobia	Sourness	Acerophobia
Points	Aichurophobia	Speaking	Halophobia
Poison	Toxiphobia	Speaking aloud	Phonophobia
Poverty	Peniaphobia	Speech	Lalophobia
Precipices	Cremnophobia	Speed	Tachophobia
		Spiders	Arachnophobia

Spirits	Demonophobia	Trees	Dendrophobia
Standing upright	Stasiphobia	Trembling	Tremophobia
Stars	Siderophobia	Tuberculosis	Phthisiophobia
Stealing	Cleptophobia	Ugliness	Dysmorephobia
Stillness	Eremophobia	Uncovering the	
Stings	Cnidophobia	body	Gymnophobia
Stooping	Kyphophobia	Vehicles	Amaxophobia
Storms	Astraphobia	Venereal disease	Cypridophobia
Strangers	Xenophobia	Void	Kenophobia
String	Linonophobia	Vomiting	Emetophobia
Sun	Heliophobia	Walking	Basiphobia
Surgical		Wasps	Spheksophobia
operations	Ergasiophobia	Water	Hydrophobia
Swallowing	Phagophobia	Weakness	Asthenophobia
Syphilis	Syphilophobia	Wind	Anemophobia
Taste	Geumatophobia	Women	Gynophobia
Teeth	Odontophobia	Words	Logophobia
Thirteen at table	Triskaidekaphobia	Work	Ergasiophobia
Thunder	Brontophobia	Worms	Helminthophobia
Thunder	Keraunophobia	Wounds, injury	Traumatophobia
Touching or		Writing	Graphophobia
being touched	Haphephobia	Young girls	Parthenophobia
Travel	Hodophobia		

REFERENCES

Abraham, G. E., and Lutran, M. M. "Serum and Red Cell Magnesium in Patients with Premenstrual Syndrome." *American Journal of Clinical Nutrition* 34 (1981): 95–103.

Abrahamson, E. M., and Peget, A. W. *Body, Mind and Sugar.* New York: Avon, 1951.

Aillon, G. A. "Biochemistry of Affective Disorders." *Psychosomatics* 12 (1971): 143–50.

Allen, A. D., and Tilkian, S. M. "Depression Correlated with Cellular Immunity in Systemic Immunodeficient Epstein-Barr Virus Syndrome (SIDES)." *Journal of Clinical Psychiatry* 47 (3) (1986): 133–135.

Alstrom, J. E., and Nordlund, C. L. "A Rating Scale for Phobic Disorders." *Acta Psychiatr. Scand.* 68 (1983): 111–16.

Arrick, C. M., and Voss, J. "The Relative Efficacy of Thought Stopping and Covert Assertion." *Behav. Res. & Ther.* 19 (1981): 17–24.

Arrindell, W. A.; Emmelkamp, P. M. G.; Brilman, E.; and Monsina, A. "Psychometric Evaluation of an Inventory for Assessment of Parental Rearing Practices." *A Dutch Form of the EMBU, Acta Psychiatrica* (1983): 34–38.

Austen, K.; Wasserman, S. I.; and Goetzel, E. J. *Molecular and Biological Aspects of the Acute Allergic Reactions.* New York: Plenum Press, 1978.

Baker, B. L.; Cohen, D. C.; and Saunders, J. T. "Self-Directed Desensitization for Agoraphobia." *Behav. Res. & Ther.* 7 (1973): 79–89.

Bakes, H., and Willis, Ursula. "School Phobic Children at Work." *Brit. J. Psychiatry* (1979): V. 135, 34–41.

Barkovec, T. D., and Robinson, E. "Preliminary Explorations of Worry: Some Characteristics and Processes." *Behav. Res. Ther.* 21 (1983): 9–16.

Barkovec, T. D., and Wilkinson, L. "Stimulus Control Applications to the Treatment of Worry." *Behav. Res. Ther.* 21 (1983): 247–51.

Barrios, B. A., and Shigetomi, C. C. "Coping Skills Training for the Management of Anxiety: A Critical Review." *Behavior Therapy* 10 (1979): 491–522.

Beisel, W. "Single Nutrient Effects on Immunological Functions." *JAMA* 245 (1981): 1246–51.

Bell, I. R. *Clinical Ecology*. Bolinas, California: Common Knowledge Press, 1982.

Bendura, A., and Reese, L. "Microanalysis of Action and Fear Arousal as a Function of Differential Levels of Perceived Self Efficacy." *Journal Pers. Social Psycho.* 43 (1982): 5–21.

Berg, I., and Fielding, D. "An Evaluation of Hospital In-Patient Treatment in Adolescent School Phobia." *British Journal of Psychiatry* 132 (1978): 500–505.

Berg, L., and Butler, A. "Psychiatric Illness in the Mothers of School Phobic Adolescents." *Br. Journal of Psychiatry* 125 (1974): 466–67.

Bergel, F. *Homeostatic Regulators*. Ciba Foundation, 1976.

Berne, Eric. *Games People Play*. New York: Grove Press, 1964.

Bernhart, M.; Gellhorn, E.; and Rasmussen, A. T. "Experimental Contributions to the Problem of Consciousness." *Journal of Neurophysiology* 19 (1953)

Bernstein, D. A. "Multiple Approaches to the Reduction of Dental Fear." *Beh. Ther. & Exp. Psychiat.* 13 (1982): 287–92.

Berygren, U., and Carlsson, S. G. "Psychometric Measures of Dental Fear." *Community Dental Orol. Epid.* 12 (1984): 319–24.

Biederman, J., and Herzoy, D. B. "Amitriptyline in the Treatment of Anorexia Nervosa: A Double-Blind, Placebo-Controlled Study." *J. of Clinical Psychopharmacology* 5 (1985): 10–13.

Blaud, Jeffery. *Nutraerobics*. San Francisco: Harper and Row, 1983.

Bolton, S. "Caffeine: Its Effects, Uses and Abuses." *Journal of Applied Nutrition* 33 (1981): 160–71.

Bomstine, P. H., and Knapp, M. "Self-Control Desensitization with a Multi-Phobic Boy: A Multiple Baseline Design." *J. Behav. Ther. & Exp. Psychiatr.* (1979): 19–20.

Bonn, J. A., and Harrison, H. "Lactate Infusion in the Treatment of Free-Floating Anxiety." *Canad. Psychiat. J.* 18 (1973): 41–45.

Borman, B. "Combat Stress, Post Traumatic Stress Disorder, Associated Psychiatric Disturbance." *Psychosomatics* 27 (1986): 567–73.

Boudoulas, H., and King, B. D. "Mitral Valve Prolapse, A Marker for Anxiety or Overlapping Phenomenon?" *Psychopathology* 7 (1983): 605–609.

Bowen, R. C. "Differential Diagnoses of Anxiety Disorders." *Prog. Neuro-Psychopharmacology and Biological Psychiat.* 7 (1983): 98–106.

Braddock, L. E. "Dysmorphophobia in Adolescence, A Case Report." *British Journal of Psychiatry* 140 (1982): 199–201.

Breznitz, S. "A Study of Worrying." *British Journal of Clin. Psychol.* 10 (1971): 271–79.

Brin, M., and Iverson, L. "Chemistry of the Brain." *Scientific American* (1980): 37–44.

Bruch, H. *Eating Disorders, Obesity, Anorexia Nervosa and Person Within.* Boston: Routledge & Kegan of America Ltd., 1974.

Brumsvels, J., and Vonderlaan, J. W. "GABA Degradation and Its Possible Relationship to the Morphine Abstinence Syndrome." *Brain Research Bull.* 5, Supp. 2 (1980): 29 797–804.

Bryce, D., and Simpson, R. I. D. "Case of Anorexia Nervosa Responding to Zinc Sulfate." *Lancet* 2 (1984): 350–84.

Buissrel, G. "Allergy." *Scientific American* 145 (1982): 77–91.

Butler, G., and Cullington, A. "Exposure and Anxiety Management in the Treatment of Social Phobias." *Journal of Consulting and Clinical Psychology* 52 (1984): 642–50.

Callahan, Roger J. *The 5-Minute Phobia Cure.* Enterprise Publishing Inc., 1985.

Cameron, E., and Pauling, L. *Cancer and Vitamin C.* New York: Norton, 1979.

Carmner, L. "Treatment of Dental Patient with Injection Phobia." *Quintessence International* 7 (1983): 759–60.

Carrera, R. N., and Lott, D. R. "The Effect of Group Implosion on Snake Phobias." *Journal of Clinical Psychology* 34 (1978): 177–80.

Casper, R. C. "Bulimia and Diet." *Archives of General Psychiatry* 3 (1980): 140–45.

Cautela, J. H. "Desensitization and Insight." *Behav. Res. Therapy* 3 (1963): 59–64.

Chaunard, G., and Labonte, A. "New Concepts in Benzodiazepine Therapy: Rebound Anxiety and New Indications for More Potent Benzodiazepines." *Prog. Neuro-Psychopharmacol. & Biol. Psychiat.* 7 (1983): 869–73.

Chen, H. C., and Hsieh, M. T. *Clinical Therapeutics* 7 (1985): 334–37.

Cheraskin, E.; Ringsdorf, W. M.; and Brescher, A. *Psychodietetics.* New York: Harper & Row, 1983.

Chernin, R. *The Obsession: Reflections on the Tyranny of Slenderness.* New York: Harper & Row, 1981.

Cobb, J., and Mathews, A. M. "The Spouse as Co-Therapist in the Treatment of Agoraphobia." *Br. J. Psychiatry* 144 (1984): 202–207.

Codie, M., and Nye, F. J. "Anxiety of Depression After Infectious Mononucleosis." *British Journal of Psychiatry* 128 (1976): 559–61.

Cohn, C. K., and Kron, R. E. "A Case of Blood-Illness-Imagery Phobia Treated Behaviorally." *Journal of Nervous and Mental Disease* 162 (1976): 65–68.

Conger, J. C., and Conger, A. J. "Fear Level as a Moderation of False Feedback Effects in Snake Phobics." *Journal of Consult. & Clin. Psychol.* 44 (1976): 133–41.

Connolly, F. H., and Gypson, M. "Dysmorphophobia—A Long Term Study." *British Journal of Psychiatry* 132 (1978): 568–70.

Coombs, R. A., and Gell, P. G. H. *Clinical Aspects of Immunology.* Oxford: Blockwell Scientific, 1968.

Coscina, D. V., and Lloyd, R. G. "Medical Hypothalamic Obesity—Association with Impaired Hypothalamic GABA Synthesis." *Brain Res. Bulletin* 5 (1980): 791–96.

Costello, C. G. "Fears and Phobias in Women, A Community Study." *Journal Abnor. Psychol.* 91 (1982): 280–86.

Crook, William G. *Tracking Down Hidden Food Allergies.* Jackson, Tennessee: Professional Books, 1978.

———. *The Yeast Connection.* Jackson, Tennessee: Professional Books, 1985.

Dahi, L. K. "Salt and Hypertension." *American Journal of Clinical Nutrition* 25 (1972): 57–61.

Dalton, Katherine. *Once a Month.* Claremont, California: Hunter House, 1979.

Dasberg, H. Shalif. "On the Validity of the Middlesex Hospital Questionnaire: A Comparison of Diagnostic Self-Ratings in Psychiatric Out Patients, General Practice Patients, and Normals Based on the Hebrew Version." *Behav., J. Med. Psychol.* 51 (1978)

Davis, P. *Nutrition Needs and Biochemical Diversity: Medical Applications of Clinical Nutrition.* New Canaan, Connecticut: Keats Pub. Co., 1983.

Deffenbacher, J. L., and Kemper, C. C. "Systemic Desensitization of Test Anxiety in Junior High Students." *School Counselor* 21 (3) (1974): 216–222.

Denney, D. R., and Sullivan, B. J. "Desensitization and Modeling Treatments of Spider Fear Using Two Types of Scenes." *Journal of Consult. & Clinical Psychology* 44 (1976): 573–79.

Dent, R. M. "Endocrine Correlates of Aggression." *Prog. Neuro-Psychopharmacol. & Biol. Psychiat.* 7 (1983): 525–28.

Denton, Derek. *The Hunger for Salt.* New York: Springer-Verlag, 1982.

Dolan, A. T., and Sheikh, A. "Short Term Treatment of Phobia Through Eidetic Imagery." *American Journal of Psychotherapy* 2 (1979): 595–605.

Donner, L. "Automated Group Desensitization: A Follow-up Report." *Behav. Res. & Therapy* 8 (1970): 241–47.

D'Orban, P. T. "Premenstrual Syndrome: A Disease of the Mind." *Lancet* (Dec. 1981): 920–26.

Dufty, W. *Sugar Blues.* Denver, Colorado: Nutri Books, 1982.

Durlock, J. "Latent Tetany Due to Chronic Magnesium Deficit and Idiopathic Mitral Valve Prolapse." *Magnesium Bull.* 1 (1981): 25–26.

Eddy, Walter H., Ph.D. *Vitaminology.* Baltimore: Williams & Wilkins, 1949.

Efran, J. S., and Archer, M. "Should Fearful Individuals Be Instructed to Proceed Quickly or Cautiously?" *Journal of Clinical Psychology* 33 (1977): 535–39.

Ellis, A. *Reason and Emotion in Psychotherapy.* New York: Stuart, 1962.

Ellis, M. E. "Evolution of Aversive Information Processing: A Temporal Tradeoff Hypothesis." *Brain Behavior* 21 (1982): 151–60.

Emmelkamp, M. G., and VonDerHout, A. "Assertive Training for Agoraphobics." *Behavioral Res. Therapy* 4 (1983): 63–68.

Emmelkamp, P. M. "Phobias." *Ned. Tydshur Geneskd* 129 (11) (1985): 489–92.

Etkin, H. "Sustained Respiratory Anxiety for Relief of a Simple Phobia." *S. A. Medical Journal* (1973): 2389–90.

Evans, P. D., and Kellam, A. M. "Semi-Automated Desensitization: A Controlled Trial." *Behavior Research Therapy* 11 (4) (1973): 641–646.

Eysenck, H. J., and Rochman, S. *The Causes and Cures of Neuroses.* San Diego, California: Knopp, 1965.

Faehton, S. *Allergy Self-Help Book.* Emmaus, Pennsylvania: Rodale Press, 1969.

Farley, F. H., and Mealien, W. L. "Sex Differences, Response Sets and Response Basis in Fear Assessment." *Journal Behav. Ther. & Exp. Psychiat.* 12 (1981): 302–32.

Faust, I. M. *The Body Weight Regulatory System.* New York: Raven Press, 1981.

Fazio, A. F. "Implosive Therapy with Semiclinical Phobias." *Journal of Abnormal Psychology* 80 (1978): 183–88.

Feingold, Benjamin. *Why Your Child Is Hyperactive.* New York: Random House, 1975.

Felice, M., and Grant, J. "Follow-Up Observations of Adolescent Rape Victims." *Clinical Pediatrics* 17 (1978): 167–70.

Ferguson, B., and Strobel, G. *Clinical Reactions to Food.* New York: Wiley & Sons, 1983.

Forbes, G. B. "Is Obesity a Genetic Disease?" *Contemporary Nutrition* 8 (1981): 73–80.

Ford, C. V. "The Somatizing Disorder." *Psychosomatics* 27 (1986): 327–37.

Forman, R. *How to Control Your Allergies.* New York: Larchmont Books, 1979.

Fox, J. "Scientists Face Explosion of Brain Compounds." *Chemical and Engineering News* 3 (Nov. 1979): 89–93.

Fox, J. E., and Houston, B. K. "Efficiency of Self-Instructional Training for Reducing Children's Anxiety in Evaluative Situations." *Behav. Res. and Therapy* 19 (1981): 509–15.

Frances, A., and Zitrin, C. M. "Treating a Man Who Cannot Go Out Alone, Feels Bound to His Ailing Mother." *Hospital Community Psychiatry* 3 (3) (1984): 225–26.

Fredricks, C. *Psycho Nutrition.* New York: Grosset & Dunlap, 1976.

Friedman, E., and Feldman, J. J. "The Public Looks at Dental Care." *Journal American Dent. Association* 57 (1958): 325–35.

Frohlich, E. D., and Torozi, R. C. "Hyperdynamic Beta Adrenergic Circulatory State." *Arch. Int. Med.* 123 (1969): 1–7.

Gabland, L. D.; Baker, S. M.; and McLellan, R. K. "Magnesium Deficiency in the Pathogenesis of Mitral Valve Prolapse." *Magnesium* 5 (1986): 165–174.

Garfinkel, P. E. "Some Recent Observations on the Pathogenesis of Anorexia Nervosa." *Canadian Journal of Psychiatry* 26 (1981): 27–33.

Garrow, J. S. *Energy Balance and Obesity in Man.* New York: Elsevier Science Pub., 1978.

Geiselman, P. L., and Norin, D. "Sugar Infusion Can Enhance Feeding." *Science* 213 (1982): 89–93.

Gelder, Michael. "Behavioral Therapy for Neurotic Disorders." *Australian and New Zealand Journal of Psychiatry* 13 (2) (1979): 103–108.

George, G. D., and Utiau, W. H. "Effect of Exogenous Estrogens on Minor Psychiatric Symptoms in Postmenopausal Women." *S. A. Medical Journal* 15 (Dec. 1973): 1–14.

Giannini, W. J., and Price, W. A. "Hyperphagia in Premenstrual Tension Syndrome." *J. Clin. Psych.* 46 (1985): 436–38.

———. "Prevalence of Mitral Valve Prolapse in Biopolar Affective Disorder." *American Journal of Psychiatry* 141 (8) (1984): 991–2.

Giles, T. R. "Probable Superiority of Behavioral Interventions, III: Some Obstacles to Findings." *J. Behav. Therapy & Exp. Psychiat.* 15 (1984): 23–26.

Glass, A. R.; Burman, K. D.; and Boehm, T. M. "Endocrine Function in Obesity." *Metabolism* 30 (1981): 794–801.

Goldfried, M. R., and Goldfried, A. P. *Helping People Change.* New York: Pergamon Press, 1980.

Goldstein, A. J., and Chambless, D. L. "A Reanalysis of Agoraphobia." *Behavioral Therapy* 9 (1978): 47–59.

Golos, N.; Goldbitz, F.; Golos, L.; and Spatz, F. *Coping with Your Allergies.* New York: Simon & Schuster, 1978.

Gothe, B. "Nicotine: A Different Approach to Treatment of Obstructive Sleep Apnea." *Chest* (1985): 7–11.

Gray, J. *The Psychology of Fear and Stress.* New York: McGraw-Hill, 1977.

Green, R. S., and Rau, J. H. *Anorexia Nervosa.* New York: Raven Press, 1977.

Greenblatt, P. J., and Shader, R. I. "On the Psychopharmacology of Beta-Adrenergic Blockage." *Current Therapy Research* 14 (1972): 615–21.

Gregory, B. A. "The Menstrual Cycle and Its Disorders in Psychiatric Patients II. Clinical Studies." *Journal of Psychosomatic Research* 2 (1957): 199–224.

Greiz, E., and VanDenHout, M. A. "The Treatment of Phobophobia by Exposure of CO_2–Induced Anxiety Symptoms." *Journal of Nervous and Mental Disease* 171 (1983): 506–8.

Gross, A. M., and Brighham, T. A. "A Comparison of Self-Delivered Consequences and Desensitization in the Treatment of Fear of Rats." *Journal of Clinical Psychology* 35 (1979): 384–90.

Gross, H. A., and Ebert, M. H. "A Double Blind Controlled Trial of Lithium Carbonate in Primary Anorexia Nervosa." *Journal of Clin. Psychopharmacal.* 1 (1981): 376–81.

Gross, M. *The Psychological Society.* New York: Simon & Schuster, 1978.

Hafner, R. J. "Agoraphobic Women Married to Abnormally Jealous Men." *British Journal of Medical Psychology* 52 (1979): 14–18.

———. "Behavioral Therapy as a Test of Psychoanalytic Theory." *Beh. Res. Therapy* 21 (1983a): 88–90.

————. "Behavioral Therapy for Agoraphobic Men." *Behav. Res. Ther.* 21 (1983b): 31–36.

Hafner, R. J., and Ross, M. W. "Predicting the Outcome of Behavior Therapy of Agoraphobia." *Beh. Res. Therapy* 21 (1983): 373–82.

Hall, R. H. *Food for Nought.* New York: Harper & Row, 1977.

Halmi, K. A. "Relationship of the Eating Disorders to Depression—Biological Similarities and Differences." *Int. J. Eating Dis.* 4 (1985): 667–80.

Hamburg, D. A. "Health and Behavior." *Science* 213 (1982): 63–70.

Hamilton, M., and Schroeder, H. E. "A Comparison of Systemic Desensitization and Reinforced Practice Procedures in Fear Reduction." *Behav. Res. & Therapy* 11 (1973): 649–52.

Hancock, J. C., and Bevilacqua, A. R. "Temporal Lobe Dysrhythmia and Impulsive or Suicidal Behavior." *Southern Medical Journal* 64 (10) (1971): 1189–93.

Hare, F. *The Food Factor in Disease.* London: Green, 1905.

Hart, K. E. "Anxiety Management Training and Anger Control for Type A Individuals." *J. Behav. Ther. & Exp. Psychiat.* 13 (1984): 133–39.

Hartman, E. "Two Case Reports: Night Terrors with Sleepwalking—A Potentially Lethal Disorder." *Journal of Nervous and Mental Disease* 171 (1983): 37–40.

————. *The Nightmare, the Psychology and Biology of Terrifying Dreams.* New York: Basic Books, 1984.

Hemmings, W. *Food Antigens and the Gut.* Berkeley: Lancaster Press, 1979.

Herman, B. P., and Chhabria, S. "Interictal Psychopathology in Patients with Fetal Fear, Examples of Sensory Limbic Hyperconnection." *Arch. Neurol.* 37 (1980): 667–68.

Hobbs, H. "Sources of Gain in Psychotherapy." *American Psychology* 17 (1962): 741–47.

Hoffer, Myron A. *Roots of Human Behavior.* San Francisco: Freeman, 1981.

Hogan, R. A., and Kirchner, J. H. "Implosion, Eclectic, Verbal and Bibliotherapy in the Treatment of the Fear of Snakes." *Behav. Res. & Therapy* 6 (1968): 167–71.

Holmi, K. A. "Catecholamine Metabolism in Anorexia Nervosa." *Int. Journal of Psychiat. Med.* 11 (1981): 251–54.

Holt, M. M. "Fear of Criticism in Washers, Checkers and Phobics." *Behav. Res. & Therapy* 17 (1979): 79–81.

Hoy, G. G. "Paranoia and Dysmorphophobia." *British Journal of Psychiatry* 142 (1983): 309–10.

Hudson, C. J., and Perkins, S. H. "Panic Disorder and Alcohol Misuse." *Journal of Studies on Alcohol* 45 (1984): 462–64.

Hudson, J., and Harrison, P. "Treatment of Bulimia with Antidepressants: Theoretical Considerations and Clinical Findings." *Psychiatric Annals* 13 (1983): 80–87.

Hunter, B. T. *The Great Nutritional Robbery.* New York: Scribner, 1978.

INC. Magazine, April 1986, pp. 53–60, Inc. Pub. Corp., Boston, Mass.

Insel, T. R. "Serotonin Blockers Seem Useful in Obsessive Compulsive Disorder." *Clinical Psychiatry News* 14 (1986): 22–28.

Iverson, T. "Neurotransmitters and Central Nervous System Disease." *Lancet* (1982): 980–81.

Jackson, H. J., and King, N. J. "The Emotive Imagery Treatment of a Child's Trauma-Induced Phobia." *J. Behavioral & Exp. Psychiatr.* 12 (1981): 325–28.

Jacobson, E. *Progressive Relaxation.* Chicago: University of Chicago Press, 1938.

Jarvis, D. C., M.D. *Folk Medicine.* New York: Henry Holt & Co., 1958.

———. *Arthritis and Folk Medicine.* New York: Fawcett, 1960.

Jellineck, E. M. *The Disease Concept of Alcoholism.* Highland Park, New Jersey: Hillhouse Pub. Co., 1960.

Johnson, C., and Stuckey, M. "Psychopharmacological Treatment of Anorexia Nervosa and Bulimia." *J. of Nervous and Mental Disease* 171 (1983): 396–400.

Johnson, D. G. "Assessment of Agoraphobia and Panic Disorder." *Prog. Neuro-Psychopharmacology and Biol. Psychiat.* 7 (1983): 617–21.

Klepac, R. K., and Dowling, J. "Characteristics of Clients Seeking Therapy for the Reduction of Dental Avoidance: Reaction to Pain." *Beh. Ther. and Exp. Psychiat.* 13 (1982): 293–300.

Klesges, R. C., and Malott, J. M. "The Effects of Graded Exposure and Parental Modeling on the Dental Phobias of a Four-Year-Old Girl and Her Mother." *J. Behav. Ther. & Exp. Psychiat.* 15 (1984): 12–14.

Klopf, H. A. *The Hedonistic Neuron Hemisphere.* London: Hemisphere, 1982.

Kolata, G. "Brain Receptors for Appetite Discovered." *Science* 218 (1982): 4.

Kolvin, J. "Aversive Imagery Treatment of Adolescents." *Behav. Res. & Therapy* 5 (1967): 245–48.

Kropf, N., and Nawas, M. M. "Standardized Scheduled Desensitization: Some Unstable Results and an Improved Program." *Beh. Res. & Therapy* 9 (1972): 35–38.

Kurnar, K., and Wilkinson, G. M. "Thought Stopping: A Useful Treatment in Phobias of Internal Stimuli." *British Journal of Psychiatry* 119 (1971): 305–7.

Kutver, S. J., and Brown, W. L. "Types of Oral Contraceptives, Depression and Premenstrual Syndrome." *Journal of Nervous and Mental Disease* 155 (1972): 153–62.

Landau, D. L., and McGlynn, F. D. "Demand Effects for Desensitization and Two Placebos in a Dental Context." *J. Behav. & Exp. Psychiat.* 15 (1984): 115–21.

Last, C. G., and Blanchard, E. B. "Classification of Phobics Versus Non-Phobics: Procedural and Theoretical Issues." *Behavioral Assess.* 4 (1982): 195–210.

Laybourne, P. C., and Redding, J. G. "Agoraphobia: Is Fear the Basis of Symptoms?" *Post Grad. Med.* 78 (1985): 109–18.

Lazarus, A. A. "Behavioral Rehearsal vs. Non-Directive Therapy vs. Advice Effective Behavior Change." *Behav. Res. & Therapy* 4 (1966): 209–12.

Leibowitz, M. R., and Kelin, D. F. "Differential Diagnoses and Treatment of Panic Attacks and Phobic States." *Ann. Rev. Med.* 32 (1981): 583–99.

Leone, C. "Thought-Induced Change in Phobic Beliefs—Sometimes It Helps, Sometimes It Hurts." *Journal of Clinical Psychology* 40 (1984): 68–71.

Lesser, M. *Nutrition and Vitamin Therapy.* New York: Grove Press, 1980.

Levenkron, S. *The Best Little Girl in the World.* New York: Warner Books, 1978.

Levine, S. *Antioxidant Biochemical Adaptation.* San Leandro, California: Biocurrents Research Corp., 1984.

Levinson, Harold N. *Phobia-Free.* New York: M. Evans, 1986.

Levitt, T. *Marketing for Business Growth.* New York: McGraw-Hill, 1969.

Lifton, R. J., and Olson, E. "The Human Meaning of Total Disaster." *Psychiatry* 38 (1976): 96–104.

Lindner, R. *The Fifty-Minute Hour.* New York: Reinhart, 1954.

Lindy, J. D., and Green, B. L. "Psychotherapy with Survivors of the Beverly Hills Supper Club Fire." *American Journal of Psychotherapy* 120 (1972): 245–58.

Lonsdale, D., and Shamberger, R. J. "Red Cell Transketolase as an Indicator of Nutritional Deficiency." *Am. Journal of Clinical Nutrition* 33 (1980): 205–11.

Lopez-Ibor, J. J. "Masked Depression." *British Journal of Psychiatry* 120 (1972): 245–58.

Luce, Gay. *Body Time.* New York: Pantheon Books, 1971.

Lydiard, R. B., and Laraia, M. T. "Can Panic Disorder Present as Irritable Bowel Syndrome?" *Journal of Clinical Psychiatry* 47 (1986): 470–73.

McConaughy, R. S. "Prognosis in Anorexia Nervosa Patient Linked with Age at Onset." *Clinical Psychiatry News* (1986): 79–82.

McDonald, T., "Effects of Visible Light Waves on Arthritis Pains." *International Journal of Biosocial Research* (1982): 233–39.

McGlynn, F. D., and Barrios, B. A. "Psychophysiological Responses to Presentation of a Caged Snake Among Behaviorally Avoidant and Non-Avoidant College Students." *Journal of Clinical Psychology* 34 (1978): 313–19.

McGlynn, F. D., and Bichanjian, C. "Effects of Cue-Controlled Relaxation, a Credible Placebo Treatment and No Treatment on Shyness Among College Males." *Journal Behav. Therapeu. & Exp. Psychiat.* 12 (1981): 299–306.

McNally, R. J., and Streketee, G. S. "The Etiology and Maintenance of Severe Animal Phobias." *Behav. Res. Ther.* 23 (1985): 431–35.

Mackomess, R. *Eating Dangerously: The Hazards of Hidden Allergies.* New York and London: Harcourt Brace Jovanovich, 1976.

MacPhail, D., and McMillan, I. "Tightening Phobias." *Nursing Mirror* (August 17, 1983): 30–33.

Magovin, H. W. *The Walking Brain.* Springfield, Illinois: Thomas, 1963.

Mandel, Marshall. *5-Day Allergy Relief Symptoms.* Pocket Books, 1980.

Marks, I., and Christopher, G. W. "Treatments of a Dentist's Phobia of Practicing Dentistry." *British Dental Journal* 147 (1979): 189–91.

Marks, I. M. *Fears and Phobics.* London: Heineman, 1969.

Marks, M., and Gray, S. "Imipramine and Brief Therapist-Aided Exposure in Agoraphobia Having Self Exposure Homework." *Arch. Gen. Psychiatry* 40 (1983): 151–61.

Martin, I. L. "The GABA-Benzodiazepine Receptor Complex." *Pro. Neuro-Pharm. & Biol. Psychiat.* 7 (1983): 433–38.

Mason, S. T., and Fibiges, H. C. "Anxiety, The Locus Disconnection." *Life's Sciences* 25 (1979): 2141–47.

Matsumi, J. T. "Taijim Kyofusho, Diagnostic and Cultural Issues in Japanese Psychiatry." *Cultural Medicine and Psychiatry* 3 (1979): 231–45.

Mavessakalian, M. "Anorexia Nervosa Treated with Response Prevention and Prolonged Exposure." *Behavior Res. Ther.* 20 (1982): 27–31.

May, J. R. "A Psychophysiological Study of Self and Externally Regulated Phobic Thought." *Behavioral Therapy* 8 (1977): 849–61.

Messtrom, M., and Cicala, G. A. "General vs. Specific Trait Anxiety Measures in the Prediction of Fear of Snakes, Heights, and Darkness." *Journal of Consult. & Clinical Psychology* 44 (1976): 83–91.

Mikkelson, E. S.; Detior, J.; and Cohen, D. S. "School Avoidance and Social Phobia Triggered by Haloperidol in Patients with Tourette's Disorder." *American Journal of Psychiatry* 138 (12) (1981): 1572–1576.

Miller, J. *Food Allergy.* Springfield, Illinois: Charles C. Thomas, Publisher, 1979.

Millman, M. *Such A Pretty Face: Being Fat in America.* New York: Berkley Press, 1980.

Milton, F., and Hafner, R. J. "The Outcome of Behavioral Therapy for Agoraphobia in Relationship to Marital Adjustment." *Arch. Gen. Psychiatry* 36 (1979): 807.

Monroe, J., and Brostoff, J. "Food Allergy in Migraine." *Lancet* 4 (1980): 1173.

Moyes, R., and Kletti, R. "Depersonalization in the Face of Life-Threatening Danger: A Description." *Psychiatry* 39 (1976): 12–14.

Mueller, P. S., and Allen, N. G. "Diagnosis and Treatment of Severe Light Sensitive Seasonal Allergy Syndrome (SES) and Its Relationship to Melatonin Anabolism." *Psychiatry Letter* (Sept. 1984): 3–4.

Mullaney, J. A., and Trippet, C. J. "Alcohol Dependence and Phobias." *Brit. J. Psychiatry* 135 (1979): 565–73.

Munjack, D. J. "The Onset of Driving Phobias." *Journal of Behavioral Therapy and Exp. Psychiat.* 15 (1984): 305–8.

Murray, E. J., and Foote, F. "The Origins of Fear of Snakes." *Behavr. Res. & Therapy* 17 (1979): 489–93.

Neese, R. M., and Cameron, O. G. "Urinary Catecholamine and Mitral Valve Prolapse in Panic-Anxiety Patients." *Psychiatry Research* 14 (1984): 67–74.

Newbolt, H. L. *Mega Nutrients for Your Nerves.* New York: Wyden Books, 1978.

Norvin, D. *Hunger, Basic Mechanisms and Clinical Implications.* New York: Raven Press, 1976.

Oda, T., and Hamamoto, K. "Effect of Coenzyme Q10 on the Stress-Induced Decrease of Cardiac Performance in Pediatric Patients With Mitral Valve Prolapse." *Jpn Circ. J.* 48 (1984): 2–3.

Orbach, S. *Fat is a Feminist Issue.* New York: Berkley Press, 1978.

Orford, J., and Edwards, G. "Abstinence or Control, the Outcome for Excessive Drinkers Two Years After Consultation." *Behav. Res. Ther.* 14 (1976): 409–18.

Orwin, A. "Respiratory Relief: A New and Rapid Method of the Treatment of Phobic States." *Brit. J. of Psychiat.* 119 (1971): 633–37.

———. "Augmented Respiratory Relief." *Brit. J. of Psychiat.* 122 (1973): 171–73.

Ost, L. G. "Fading: A New Technique in the Treatment of Phobias." *Beh. Res. & Therapy* 16 (1978): 213–16.

———. "Fading vs. Systematic Desensitization in the Treatment of Snake and Spider Phobia." *Behav. Res. and Therapy* 16 (1978): 379–89.

Ost, L. G., and Jerremalm, A. "Individual Response Patterns and the Effects of Different Behavioral Methods in the Treatment of Social Phobias." *Beh. Res. Therp.* 19 (1981): 1–16.

Ost, L. G., and Sterner, U. "Physiological Responses in Blood Phobics." *Beh. Res. Therp.* 22 (1984): 109–17.

Ott, J. *Light and Health.* New York: Bantam Books, 1977.

Page, L., and Friend, B. "The Changing U.S. Diet." *Bioscience* 28 (1978): 40–45.

Palfreyman, M. G.; Schecter, P. J.; and Buckett, W. R. "The Pharmacology of GABA Transaminase Inhibitors." *Biochemical Pharmacology* 30 (1981): 817–24.

Parenteal, P., and Larmorrtagne, Y. "The Thought Stopping Technique. A Treatment of Ruminations?" *Can. Journal of Psychiatry* 26 (1981): 12–19.

Perinpanayagam, K. S. "A Monosymptomatic Phobia Treated by a Single Session of Behavioral Therapy." *Brit. J. Psychiat.* 119 (1971): 309–10.

Perls, F. *Ego, Hunger and Aggression.* New York: Random House, 1969.

Peters, R. A., and Thompson, R. H. S. "Pyruvic Acid as an Intermediary Metabolite in the Brain Tissue of Avitaminous and Normal Pigeons." *Biochemical Journal* 28 (1934): 917–25.

Philippopoulos, G. S. "The Analysis of a Case of Dysmorophobia." *Canadian Journal of Psych.* 24 (1979) 397–401.

Phillips, R. E., and Johnson, G. D. "Case Histories and Shorter Communications, Self-Administered Systemic Desensitizations." *Behav. Res. & Therapy* 10 (1972): 93–96.

Philpott, W. H., and Kalita, B. K. *Brain Allergies.* New Canaan, Connecticut: Keats Pub., 1980.

Picknold, J. C., and McLure, D. J. "Does Tryptophan Potentiate Clomipramine in the Treatment of Agoraphobia and Social Phobic Patients?" *Br. J. Psychiatry* 140 (1982): 484–90.

Pike, R., and Brown, M. *Nutrition—An Integrated Approach.* New York: Wiley, 1967.

Pitts, F. N., and Allen, R. E. *Phenomenology and Treatment of Anxiety.* New York: Spectrum Publications, 1979.

Praisner, S. B. "Disorders of Glutamate Metabolism and Neurological Dysfunction." *Amer. Rev. Med.* 32 (1981): 531–42.

Price, W. A., and Giannini, A. J. "Verapamil in the Treatment of Premenstrual Syndrome: Case Report." *J. Clin. Psychiat.* 47 (1986): 213–14.

Pull, C. B., and Overall, J. E. "Adequacy of the Brief Psychiatric Rating Scale for Distinguishing Lesser Forms of Psychopathology." *Psychological Reports* 40 (1977): 167–73.

Rakoff, V. "Children and Families of Concentration Camp Survivors." *Canada's Mental Health* 14 (1966): 24–26.

Randolph, T. G., M. D. *Human Ecology and Susceptibility to the Chemical Environment.* Springfield, Illinois: Thomas, 1962.

Randolph, T. G., and Moss, R. W. *An Alternative Approach to Allergies.* New York: Lippincott & Crowell, 1979.

Rapp, D. J. *Allergies and the Hyperactive Child.* New York: Sovereign, 1979.

Rea, W. D. "Environmentally Triggered Cardiac Disease." *Annals of Allergy* 40 (1986): 243–251.

Redmond, E. E., and Huang, Y. N. "New Evidence for a Locus Coeruleus-Norepinephrine Connection with Anxiety." *Life's Sciences* 25 (1979): 2149–62.

Richardson, S. S., and Kelinknecht, R. A. "Expectancy Effects on Anxiety and Self-Generated Cognitive Strategies in High and Low Dental-Anxious Females." *J. Behav. Ther. & Exp. Psychiat.* 15 (1984): 241–47.

Rippere, V. "Food Additives and Hyperactive Children: A Critique of Conners." *Brit. J. of Clinical Psychology* 22 (1983): 19–32.

Robimer, C. J. "Imipramine Treatment of School Phobias." *Comp. Psychiatry* 10 (1969): 387–90.

Robinson, H. "Review of Child Molestation and Alleged Rape Cases." *American Journal of Obstet. Gyn.* 110 (1971): 405.

Ross, J. "The Use of Former Phobics in the Treatment of Phobias." *American Journal of Psychiatry* 137 (1980): 715–17.

Rouch, P. K., and Stern, D. "Life-Threatening Injuries Resulting from Sleepwalking and Night Terrors." *Psychosomatics* 27 (1986): 62–64.

Rude, R. K., and Singer, F. R. "Magnesium Deficiency and Excess." *Ann. Rev. Med.* 32 (1981): 243–59.

Sartory, G., and Rochman, S. "Return of Fear: The Role of Rehearsal." *Behav. Res. Ther.* 20 (1982): 123–33.

Schauss, A. *Diet, Crime and Delinquency.* Berkeley, California: Parker House, 1981.

Schroeder, H. A. *Trace Elements and Man.* Old Greenwich, Connecticut: Devon Adair, 1973.

Schwartz, L. S., and Val, E. R. "Agoraphobia, a Multimodal Treatment Approach." *American Journal of Psychotherapy* 38 (1984): 35–46.

Scrigner, C. B., and Swenson, W. C. "Use of Systemic Desensitization in the Treatment of Phobias." *American Journal of Psychiatry* 137 (1980): 715–17.

Selye, H. *Stress.* Montreal, Canada: Acta, 1950.

Shahied, I., PhD. *Biochemistry of Foods and Biocatalysts.* New York: Vantage Press, 1980.

Shapiro, D. H., and Giver, D. "Meditation and Psychotherapeutic Effects." *Arch. Gen. Psychiatry* 35 (1978): 294–302.

Sheinkin, D.; Schacter, M.; and Hutton, R. *Food, Mind and Mood.* New York: Warner Books, 1980.

Shine, K. I. "Anxiety in Patients with Heart Disease." *Psychosomatics* 25 (1984): 127–31.

Siegel, L. J., and Peterson, L. "Stress Reduction in Young Dental Patients Through Coping Skills and Sensory Information." *Journal of Consul. & Clinical Psychol.* 48 (1980): 785–87.

Sitaram, N., and Duke, S. "Acetylcholine and A-Adrenergic Sensitivity in the Separation of Depression Anxiety." *Psychopathology* 17, Supp. 3 (1984): 24–39.

Skolinck, P., and Ninan, P. "A Novel Chemically Induced Animal Model of Human Anxiety." *Psychopathology* 17, Supp. 1 (1984): 25–26.

Slater, S. L., and Leacy, A. "The Effects of Inhaling a 35 Percent CO_2 65 Percent Mixture O_2 Upon Anxiety Level in Neurotic Patients." *Beh. Res. & Therapy* 4 (1966): 309–16.

Sloan, S. *Nutritional Parenting.* New Canaan, Connecticut: Keats Pub., 1982.

Smith, L. H. *Foods for Healthy Kids.* New York: McGraw-Hill, 1981.

Sochar, E., M.D. *Topics in Psychoendocrinology.* New York: Grune & Stratton, 1975.

Spiller, G. A. *Nutrition Pharmacology.* New York: Alan R. Liss, 1982.

Sreenivasan, U., and Manocha, S. N. "Treatment of Severe Dog Phobia in Childhood by Flooding." *Journal of Child Psychol. Psychiat.* 20 (1979): 225–60.

Stan, H. J., and McGrath, P. A. "The Treatment of Temporomandibular Joint Syndrome Through Control of Anxiety." *Journal of Behavioral Therapy & Exp. Psychiatry* 15 (1984): 41–45.

Stern, R. S., and Lipsedge, M. S. "Obsessional Ruminations: A Controlled Trial of Thought Stopping Technique." *Behav. Res. & Therapy* 11 (1973): 659–62.

Stevenson, M. "Food Allergies and Migraine." *Lancet* 121 (1979): 941.

Stotsky, B. A., and Borzne, J. "Butasol Sodium vs. Librium Among Geriatric and Younger Outpatients and Nursing Home Patients." *Diseases of the Nervous System* (1972): 254–56.

Strass, B., and Schulthess, M. "Autonomic Reactivity in the Premenstrual Phase." *British Journal of Clinical Psychology* 22 (1983): 1–9.

Surwit, R. S. "Behavioral Treatment of Raynaud's Syndrome in Peripheral Vascular Disease." *Journal of Consulting and Clinical Psychology* 50 (1982): 922–32.

Taylor, J. W. "Psychological Factors in the Aetiology of Premenstrual Symptoms." *Australian and New Zealand Journal of Psychiatry* 13 (1979): 44–50.

Telch, M. J., and Tearman, B. A. "Anti-Depressant Medication in the Treatment of Agoraphobia, A Critical Review." *Behavioral Res. Therapy* 21 (1983): 505–17.

Thompson, C. J., Ph.D. *Controls of Eating.* Jamaica, NY: Spectrum Publications, 1980.

Thyer, B. A., and Curtis, G. C. "On the Diphasic Nature of Vaso-Vagal Fainting Associated with Blood-Injury-Illness Phobia." *Pav. J. Beh. of Biological Science* 20 (1983): 84–87.

Tolbert, L. C.; Thomas, T. N.; and Middaugh, L. D. "Effects of Ascorbic Acid on Neurochemical, Behavioral and Physiological Systems Medicated by Cate-cholamine." *Life's Sciences* 25 (1979): 2189–95.

Tyrer, P., and Owen, R. T. "The Brief Scale for Anxiety: A Subdivision of the Com-prehensive Psychopathological Rating Scale." *Journal of Neurology, Neuro-surgery and Psychiatry* 47 (1984): 970–75.

Vellucci, S. A., "Studies on the Role of ACTH and of 5-HT in Anxiety, Using an Animal Model." *J. Pharm. Pharmac.* 30 (1978): 105–10.

Venhom, L. "The Effect of Mother's Presence on Child's Response to Dental Treat-ment." *Journal of Dentistry for Children* (1979): 219–24.

Vincent, L. S., M.D. *Competing with the Sylph.* Kansas City, Missouri: Andrews & McNeel, 1979.

Vose, Ruth Hearst. *Agoraphobia.* London: Faber and Faber, 1981.

Wadden, T. A., and Gister, G. D. "Self-Concept and Normal Weight Children." *Journal of Consulting and Clinical Psychology* 52 (1984): 1104–5.

Watson, J. P., and Gaind, R. "Prolonged Exposure: A Rapid Treatment for Phobias." *British Medical Journal* 9 (1971): 13–18.

Watson, J. P., and Mullett, G. E. "The Effects of Prolonged Exposure to Phobic Situations upon Agoraphobic Patients Treated in Groups." *Behav. Res. & Ther-apy* 11 (1973): 331–45.

Webster, D. R., and Azri, N. H. "Required Relaxation: A Method of Inhibiting Agitative-Disruptive Behavior of Retardates." *Behavioral Res. and Therapy* 11 (1973): 67–68.

Weil, A. A. "Ictal Depression and Anxiety in Temporal Lobe Disorders." *Am. J. of Psychiatry* 113 (1956): 149–57.

———. "Ictal Emotions Occurring in Temporal Lobe Dysfunctions." *Arc. of Neurol.* 1 (1959): 101–11.

Westphal, C. "Die Agoraphobia Eine Neuropathische Erscheinung." *Arch. Fur Psy-chiatria Und Nerven Krankheiten* 3 (1871): 138–71.

Whatmore, G. B. *Tension in Medicine.* Springfield, Illinois: Thomas, 1967.

Whatmore, G. B., and Kohli, D. "Dysponesis. A Neurophysiologic Factor in Functional Disorders." *Behavioral Science* 13 (1968): 102–24.

———. *The Physiopathology and Treatment of Functional Disorders.* New York: Grune & Stratton, 1974.

Wieselberg, N., and Dyckman, J. M. "The Desensitization Derby." *Journal of Clinical Psychology* 35 (1979): 647–50.

Williams, J. "Iron Deficiency Treatment." *Western Journal of Medicine* 1 (1981): 230–32.

Williams, R. J. *Nutrition Against Disease.* New York: Bantam Books, 1973.

Wohler, R. G., and Winkler, G. H. "Mothers as Behavioral Therapists for Their Own Children." *Behavioral and Research Therapy* 3 (1965): 113–24.

Wolpe, J., M.D. *The Practice of Behavioral Therapy.* New York: Pergamon Press, 1969.

Wolpe, Joseph. *Psychotherapy by Reciprocal Inhibition.* Stanford, California: Stanford University Press, 1958.

Wright, F. A. C., and Lange, D. E. "The Management of Dental Phobia." *New Zealand Dental Journal* 74 (1970): 210–14.

Wunderlich, R., and Kolita, D. *Candidia and the Human Condition.* New Canaan, Connecticut: Keats Pub., 1984.

Wunderlich, R. C. *Sugar and Your Health.* St. Petersburg, Florida: Good Health Pub., 1982

Wurtman, J. J., and Zeisel, S. H. "Carbohydrate Cravings in Obese People." *International Journal of Eating Disorders* 5 (1982): 45–48.

Wurtman, R. J. "Nutrients that Modify Brain Functions." *Scientific American* 2 (1982): 145–57.

Zamm, A. V., and Gannon, R. *Why Your House May Endanger Your Health.* New York: Simon & Schuster, 1980.

Zarr, M. L. "Computer Mediated Psychotherapy: Toward Patient-Selection Guidelines." *Amer. J. of Psychotherapy* 38 (1984): 13–21.

Zitron, C. M.; Klein, D. F.; and Woerner, M. G. "Behavior Therapy, Supportive Psychotherapy Imipramine and Phobias." *Archives of General Psychiatry* (1978): 307–316.

(No author given). "The Treatment of Premenstrual Symptoms." *British Journal of Psychiatry* 135 (1979): 576–79.

A PLACE TO FIND HELP

The National Self-Help Clearinghouse maintains an up-to-date listing of most mutual-aid organizations throughout the nation. You will need to send a stamped self-addressed envelope.

> *National Self-Help Clearinghouse*
> City University of New York
> 33 West 42nd St.
> New York, New York 10036
> 212-840-1259

Local numbers for support groups:

	Self Help
CALIFORNIA	800-222-LINK
CONNECTICUT	203-789-7645
ILLINOIS	312-328-0470
KANSAS	316-686-1205
MICHIGAN	616-983-7781
MINNESOTA	612-925-0585
NEBRASKA	402-476-9668
NEW JERSEY	201-625-9565
NEW YORK STATE	518-695-3418
NEW YORK CITY	212-788-8787
OHIO	216-696-4262
OREGON	503-222-5555
PENNSYLVANIA	213-568-0890 Ext. 266
TENNESSEE	615-588-9747
TEXAS	214-871-2420
WASHINGTON, D.C.	703-536-4100
WISCONSIN	414-458-0891

CALIFORNIA

Stewart W. Agras, M.D.
Department of Psychiatry
Stanford University Medical
  School
40 Parnassus Ave.
Stanford, CA 94305
(415) 723-6643

Mardi J. Horowitz, M.D.
Department of Psychiatry
Langely Porter
  Neuropsychiatric Institute
University of California
San Francisco, CA 94143
(415) 476-7000

Hunt Medical Group
3808 Riverside Drive
North Hollywood, CA 91602
(818) 840-8322

Dennis J. Munjack, M.D.
Anxiety Disorder Clinic
University of Southern
  California Medical Center
Department of Psychiatry
1937 Hospital Place
Los Angeles, CA 90033
(213) 226-5329

Terrap Panic Treatment
Program
1010 Doyle St.
Menlo Park, CA 94025
(415) 329-1233

DISTRICT OF COLUMBIA

Dianne L. Chambless, Ph.D.
Agoraphobia Program

The American University
Department of Psychiatry
Massachusetts & Nebraska
  Ave., NW
Washington, DC 20016
(202) 885-1715

FLORIDA

Carl Eisdoufer, M.D.
University of Miami
Phobia & Anxieties Clinic
1500 N.W. 12th Ave.
Miami, FL 33136
(305) 547-6755

David Sheehan, M.D.
Department of Psychiatry
University of Southern Florida
3515 E. Fletcher Ave.
Tampa, FL 33613
(813) 972-7070

GEORGIA

Phillip Ninan, M.D.
Emory University Mental Health
  Clinic
1365 Clifton Rd.
Atlanta, GA 30322
(404) 321-0111

ILLINOIS

Harry Trusman, M.D., Chm.
Department of Psychiatry
University of Chicago School of
  Medicine
5841 S. Marylon
Chicago, IL 60637
(312) 962-6181

IOWA

Russell Noyes, Jr., M.D.
Department of Psychiatry
University of Iowa School of
  Medicine
500 Newton Rd.
Iowa City, IA 52242
(319) 356-1355

MAINE

Geoffrey L. Thorpe, Ph.D.
Anxiety Disorders Research
  Program
Psychology Department
University of Maine at Orono
301 Little Hall
Orono, ME 04469
(207) 581-2055

MARYLAND

Richard Perlmutter, M.D., Dir.
Agoraphobia Treatment
  Program
Sheppard Pratt Hospital
6501 N. Charles St.
Towson, MD 21204
(301) 823-8200, Ext. 3710

MASSACHUSETTS

Richard Shader, M.D., Chm.
Tufts University Department of
  Psychiatry
750 Washington St.
Boston, MA 02111
(617) 956-5772

MICHIGAN

George Curtis, M.D.
University of Michigan Anxiety
  Disorder Program
Department of Psychiatry
University Hospital
1405 E. Ann St.
Ann Arbor, MI 48109
(313) 764-5348

Daniel Gershon, M.D.
Wayne State University School
  of Medicine
5050 Cass Ave.
Detroit, MI 48202
(313) 577-2424

John Rainey, M.D.
Lafayette Clinic
951 E. Lafayette St.
Detroit, MI 48207
(313) 256-9533

MISSISSIPPI

Edgar Draper, M.D., Chm.
University of Mississippi
  Medical Center
2500 North State St.
Jackson, MS 39216
(601) 984-5800

MISSOURI

Robert Cloniger, M.D.
Department of Psychiatry
The Jewish Hospital of St. Louis
Washington University Medical
  Center

216 South Kingshighway
P.O. Box 14109
St. Louis, MO 63178
(314) 454-8560

C. Alec Pollard, Ph.D.
1221 S. Grand Blvd.
St. Louis, MO 63104
(314) 771-6400, Ext. 202

Marcus Raichle, M.D.
Washington University School
    of Medicine
No. 1 Brookings Dr.
St. Louis, MO 63119
(314) 889-5000

NEW YORK

David H. Barlow, Ph.D., Dir.
Phobia and Anxiety Disorders
    Clinic
State University of New York at
    Albany
1535 Western Ave.
Albany, NY 12203
(518) 456-4127

Donald Klein, M.D.
New York State Psychiatric
    Institute
722 West 168 St.
New York, NY 10032
(212) 960-2366

Manuel D. Zane, M.D.
Phobic Clinic
White Plains Hospital Medical
    Center
Davis Ave. at East Rd.
White Plains, NY 10601
(914) 681-1038

PENNSYLVANIA

Alan Goldstein, Ph.D.
Agoraphobia and Anxiety
    Program of Temple
    University Medical School
Department of Psychiatry
112 Bala Ave.
Bala Cynwyg, PA 19004
(215) 667-6490

Samuel M. Turner, Ph.D.
Department of Psychiatry
University of Pittsburgh Medical
    School
Western Pennsylvania
    Psychiatric Institute
3811 O'Hara St.
Pittsburgh, PA 15261
(412) 624-1000

TENNESSEE

Roy J. Mathew, M.D.
Department of Psychiatry,
    A-2215
Medical Center North
Vanderbilt University School of
    Medicine
21st and Garland Ave.
Nashville, TN 37232
(615) 327-7009

WISCONSIN

Bela H. Selan, M.S.
Mt. Sinai Medical Center
Department of Psychiatry
950 North 125th St.
Milwaukee, WI 53233
(414) 289-8150 or 298-8620

You can write to the Phobia Society of America for a complete list of anxiety and panic disorder treatment centers.

> *Phobia Society of America*
> 133 Rollins Ave.
> Rockville, MD 20852-4004
> (301) 231-9350

You might also write to the following organization for the names of those who practice behavioral therapy in your area:

Association for
  Advancement of
  Behavioral
  Therapy
420 Lexington Ave.
New York, NY 10016

Nutritional
  Supplements

GABA Powder
  (Gamma-
  Aminobutyric Acid)
Vitamin Research
  Products
2044 Old Middlefield
  Way
Mountain View, CA 94043
800-541-1623

RESCUE
Ellon Bach, U.S.A.
P.O. Box 320
Woodmere, NY 11598

Selenium
Nutra-Cology, Inc.
Dr. Steven Levine
P.O. Box 489
400 Preda Street
San Leandra, CA 94577-0489
(415) 639-4572

Mintran
Standard Process Labs
P.O. Box 652
Milwaukee, Wisconsin 53201

Nutra-Homo
Nutra-Homo, Inc.
Los Alamitos, California

Vitamin Research
  now has 100 mg.
  sublingual GABA
  tablets for anxiety

INDEX